MAZES

Dedication

To my patients, whose courage, resilience, and trust inspire me every day. This book is dedicated to you, with gratitude for the lessons you have taught me about perseverance, healing, and the power of the human spirit. It is an honor to be a part of your story.

To my husband, family and friends, for your unwavering love, support and encouragement in all my endeavors. You are priceless.

And mostly, to my Lord and Savior, Jesus Christ.

With much love,
Laura

About the Author

With a dedication to healthcare innovation and patient focused care, Laura has served patients for over 29 years and has a distinguished career in the field of speech-language pathology and home health care. As one of the founders of a CHAP accredited, Medicare certified home health agency, she achieved recognition by HomeCare Elite as one of the top 25% of certified home health agencies nationwide in 2012, 2014, 2015 and 2016. Additionally, Laura led a private pay personal care agency to generate over $1.5 million in revenue within the first 18 months of its inception, exemplifying a commitment to quality and service.

Laura holds both a Masters of Science degree in Speech Pathology and Audiology and a Bachelor of Arts degree from Baylor University, with specialized certifications including Vital Stimulation and Lee Silverman Voice Treatment. This clinical expertise, coupled with extensive experience in healthcare management, is central to Laura's therapy approach to serving her patients. Laura remains licensed to practice by State Board of Examiners for Speech Language Pathology and Audiology and holds the Certificate of Clinical Competence with the American Speech Language and Hearing Association (ASHA).

Maze #1

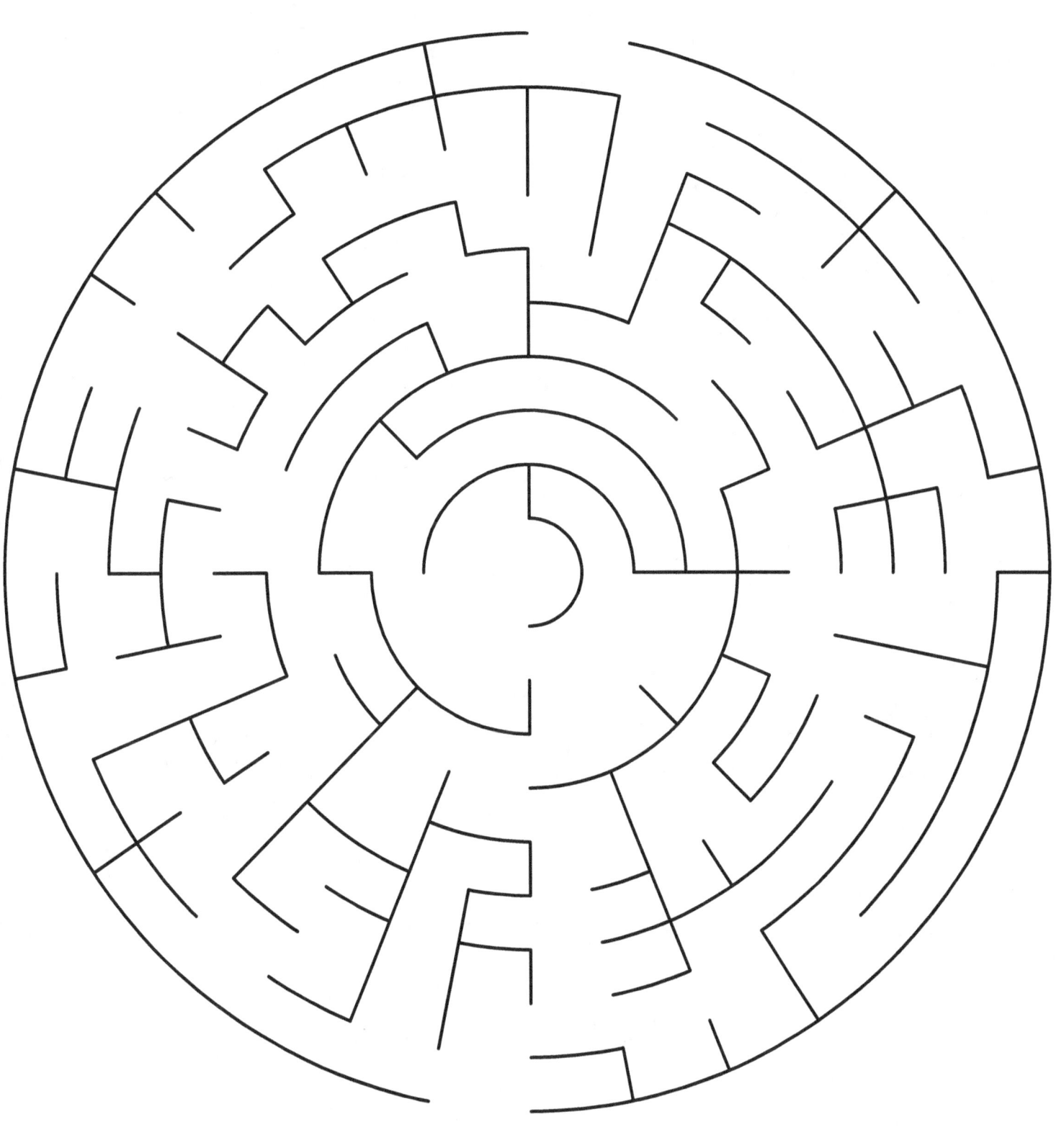

Maze #2

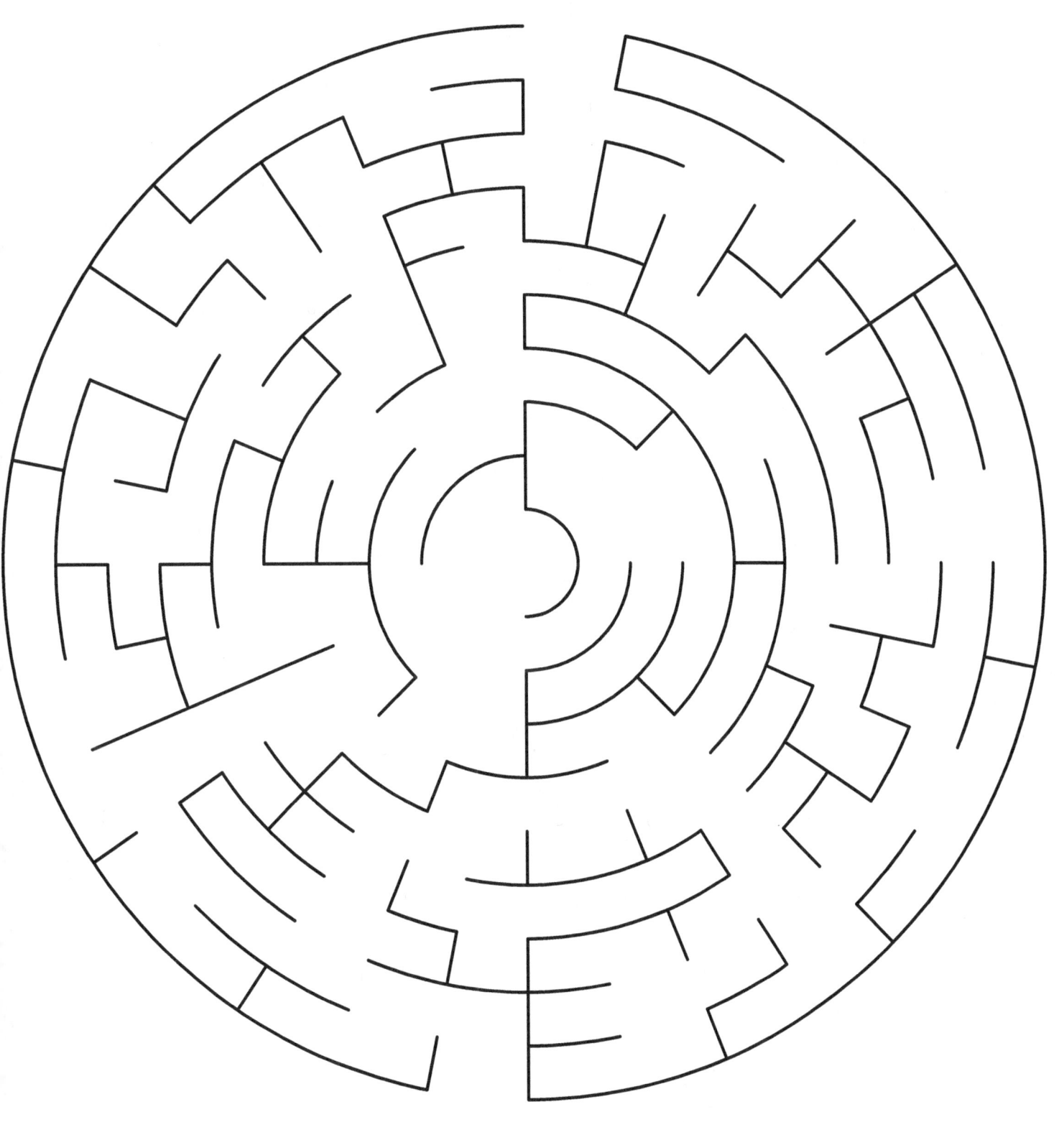

Maze #3

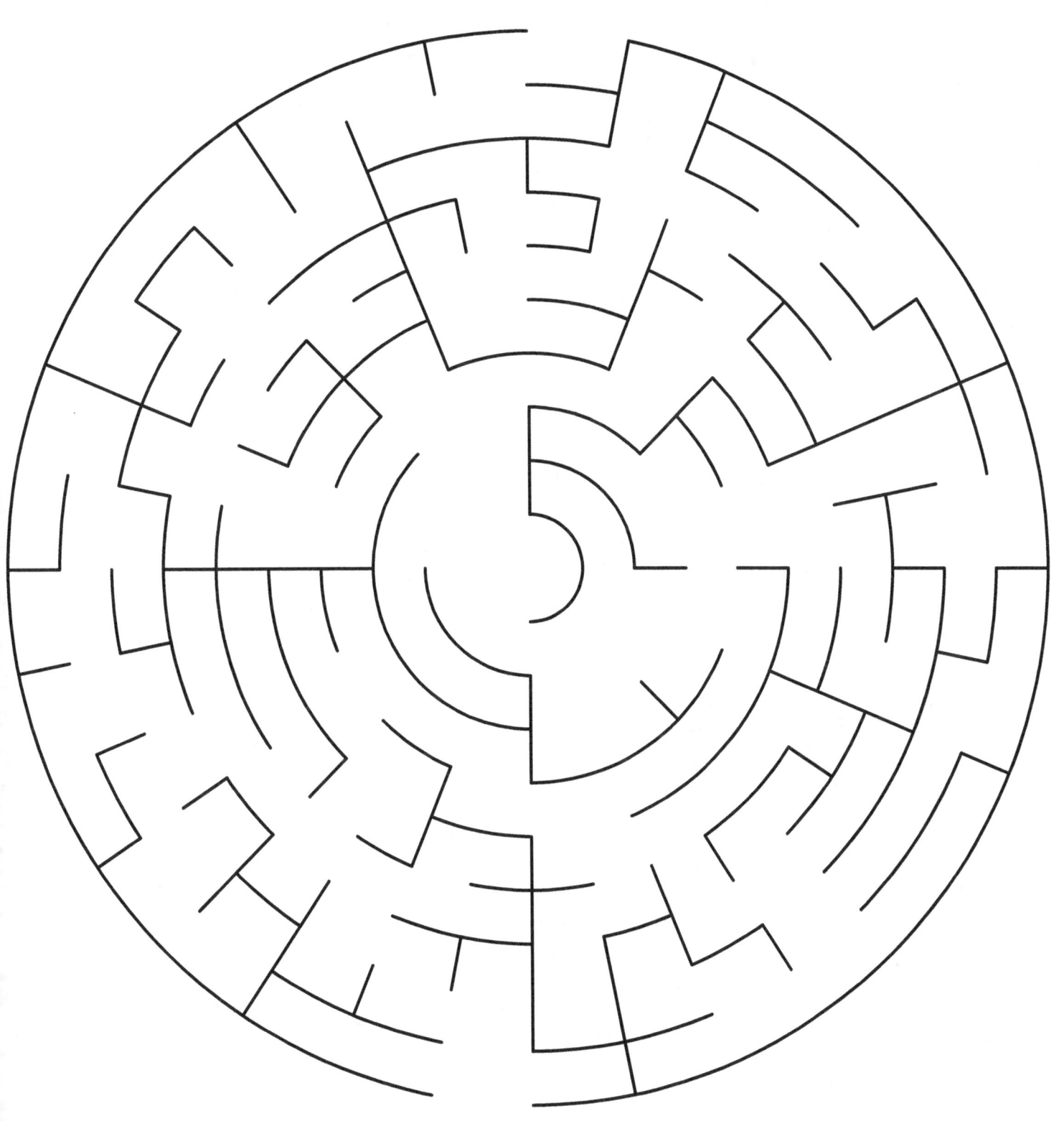

Maze #4

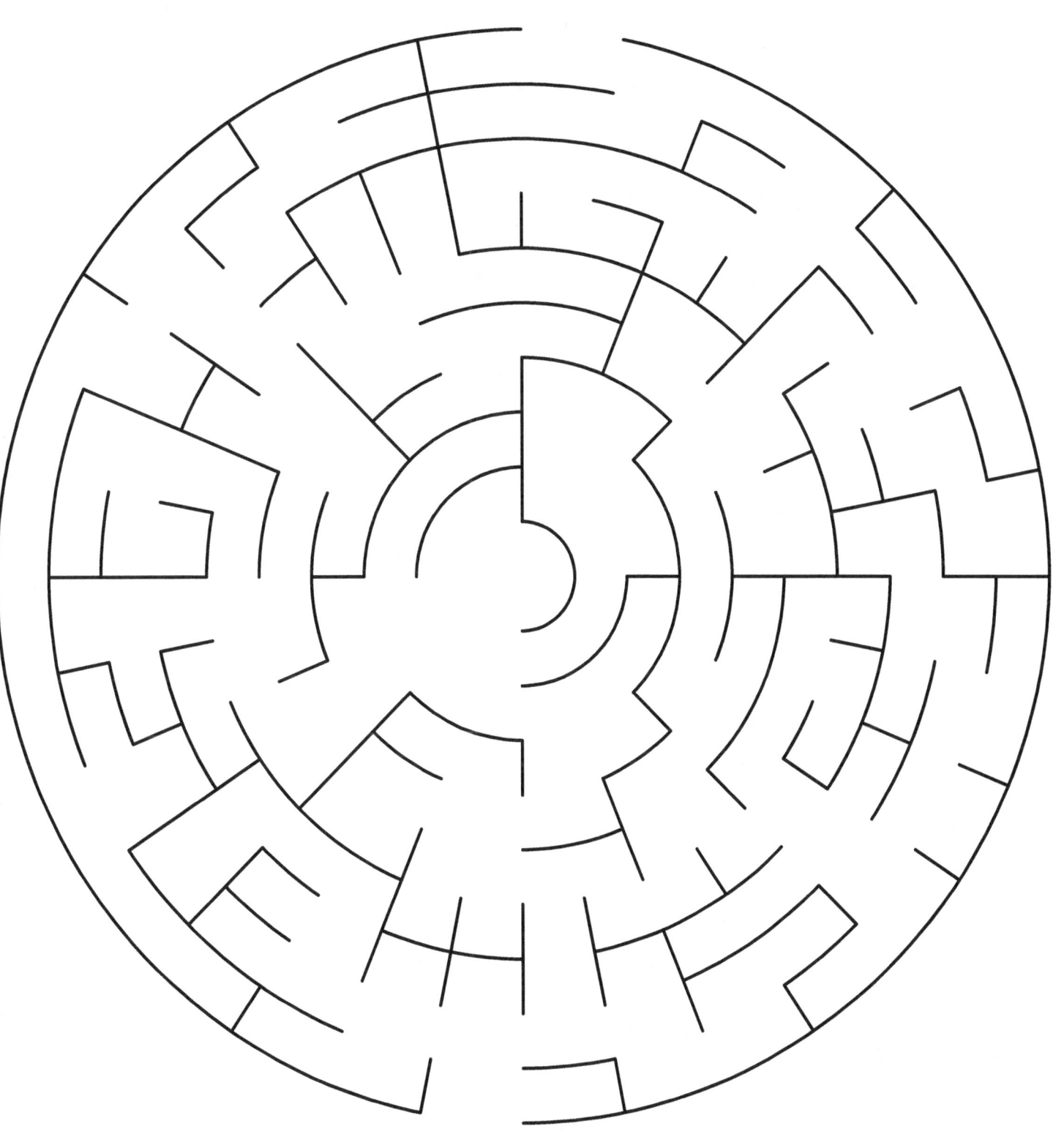

Maze #5

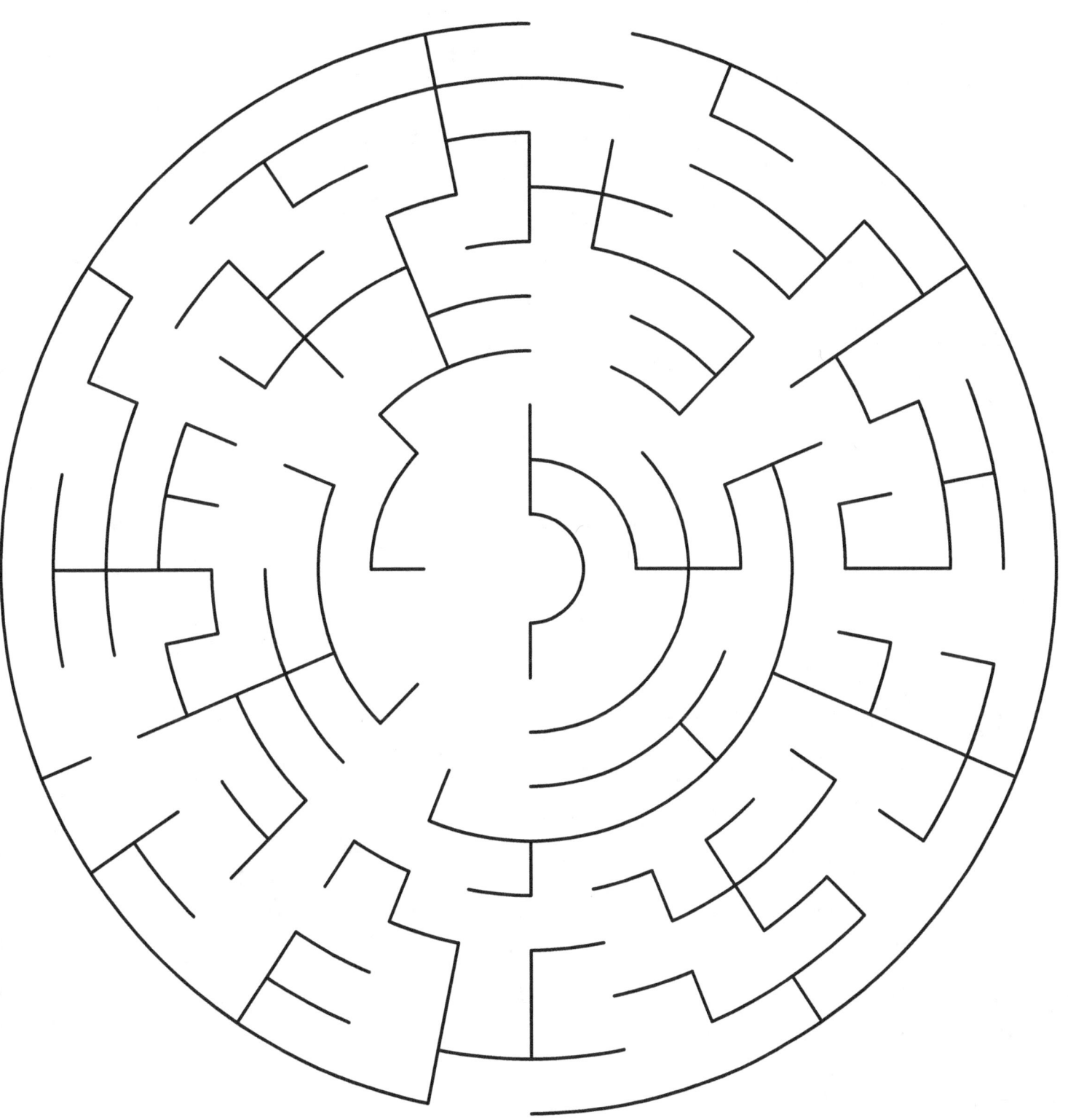

Maze #6

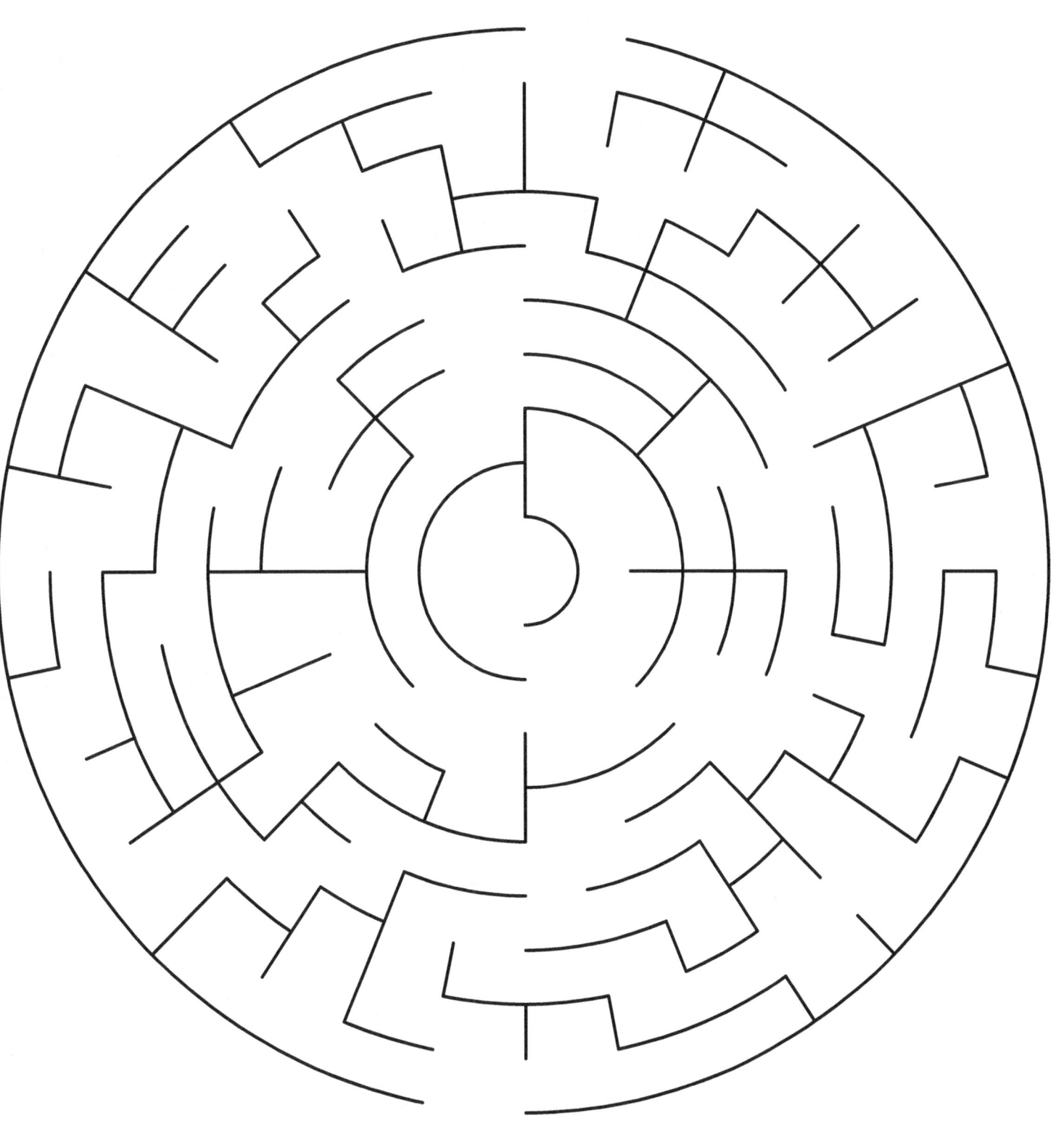

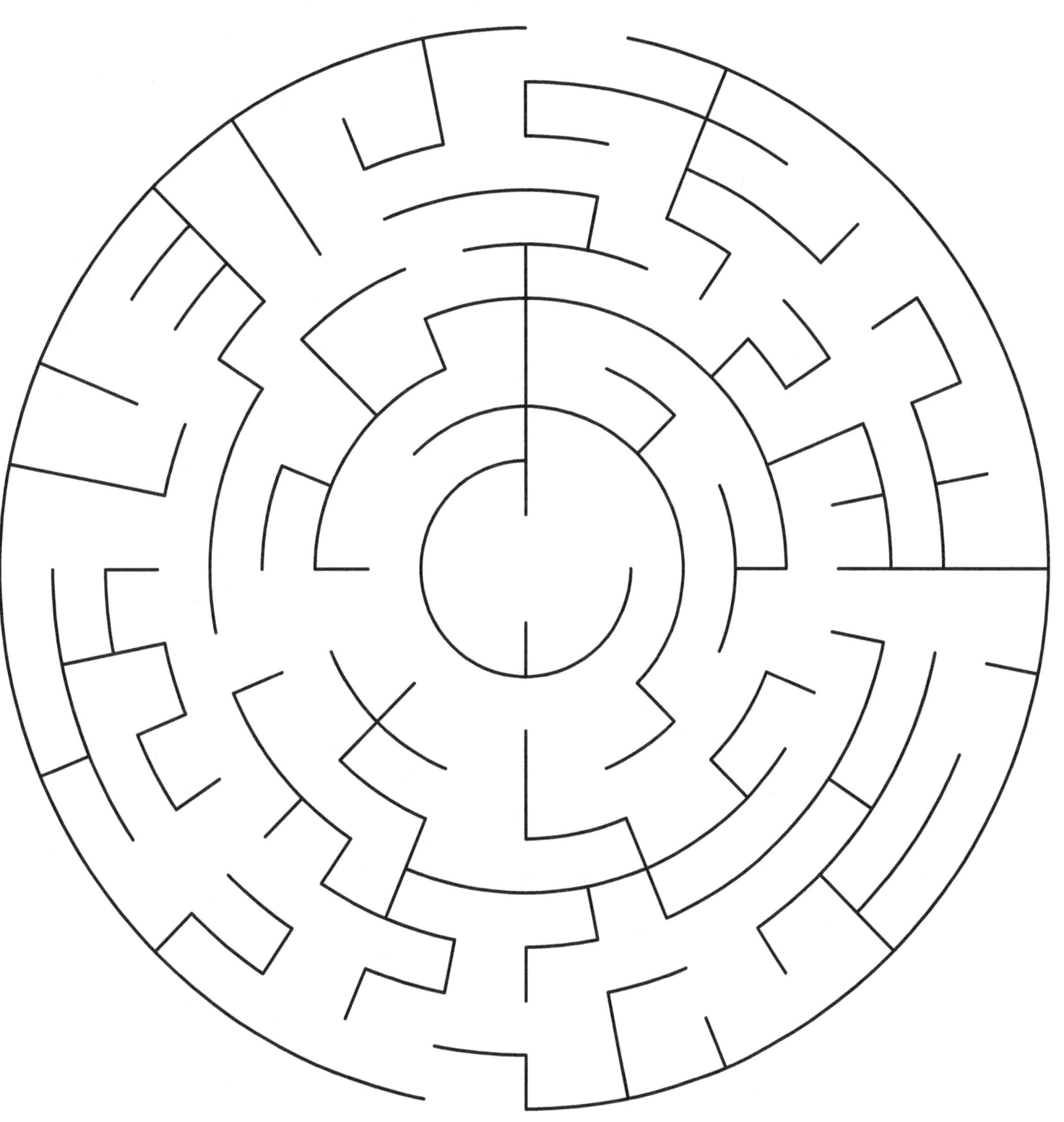

Maze #8

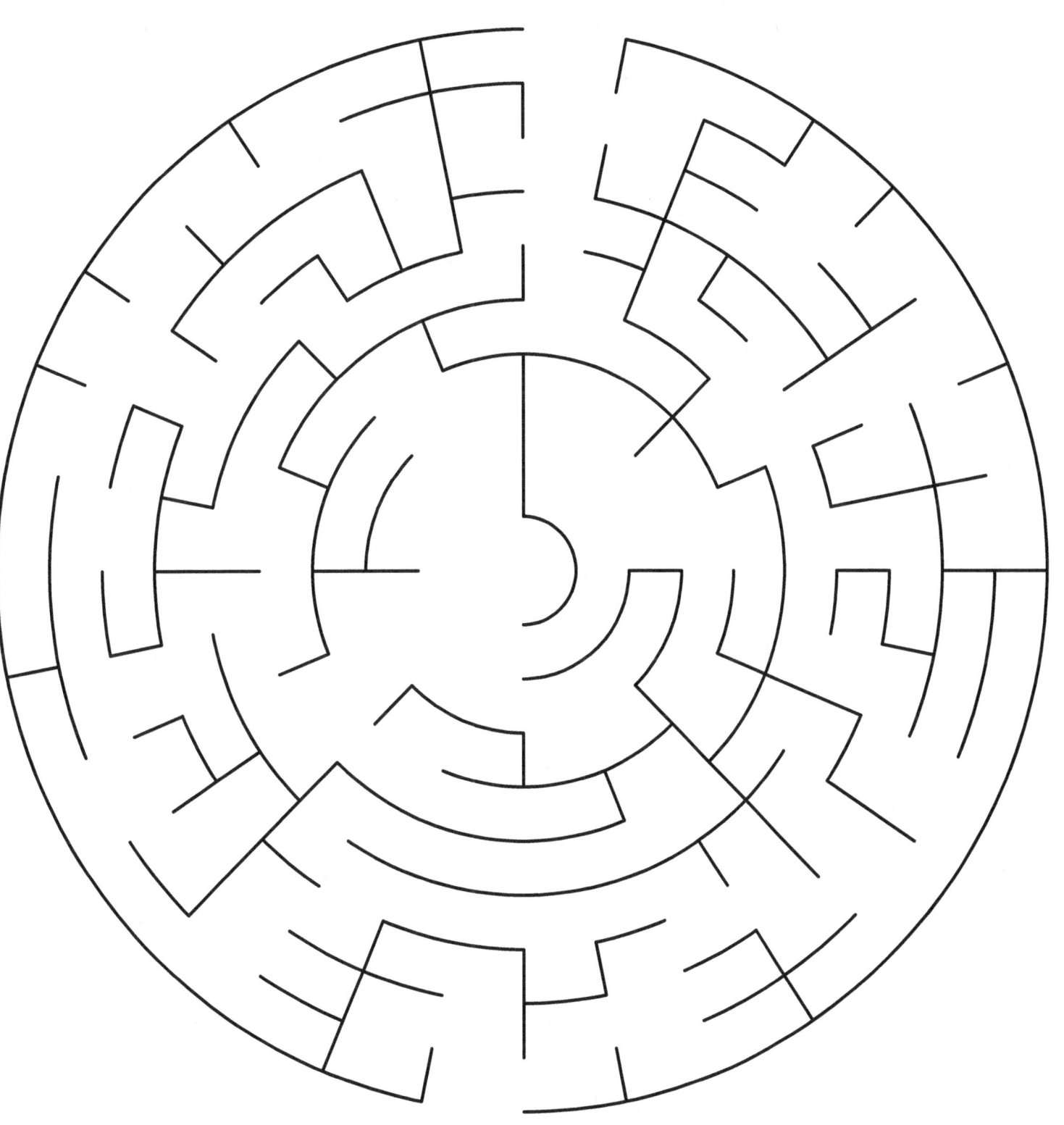

Maze #9

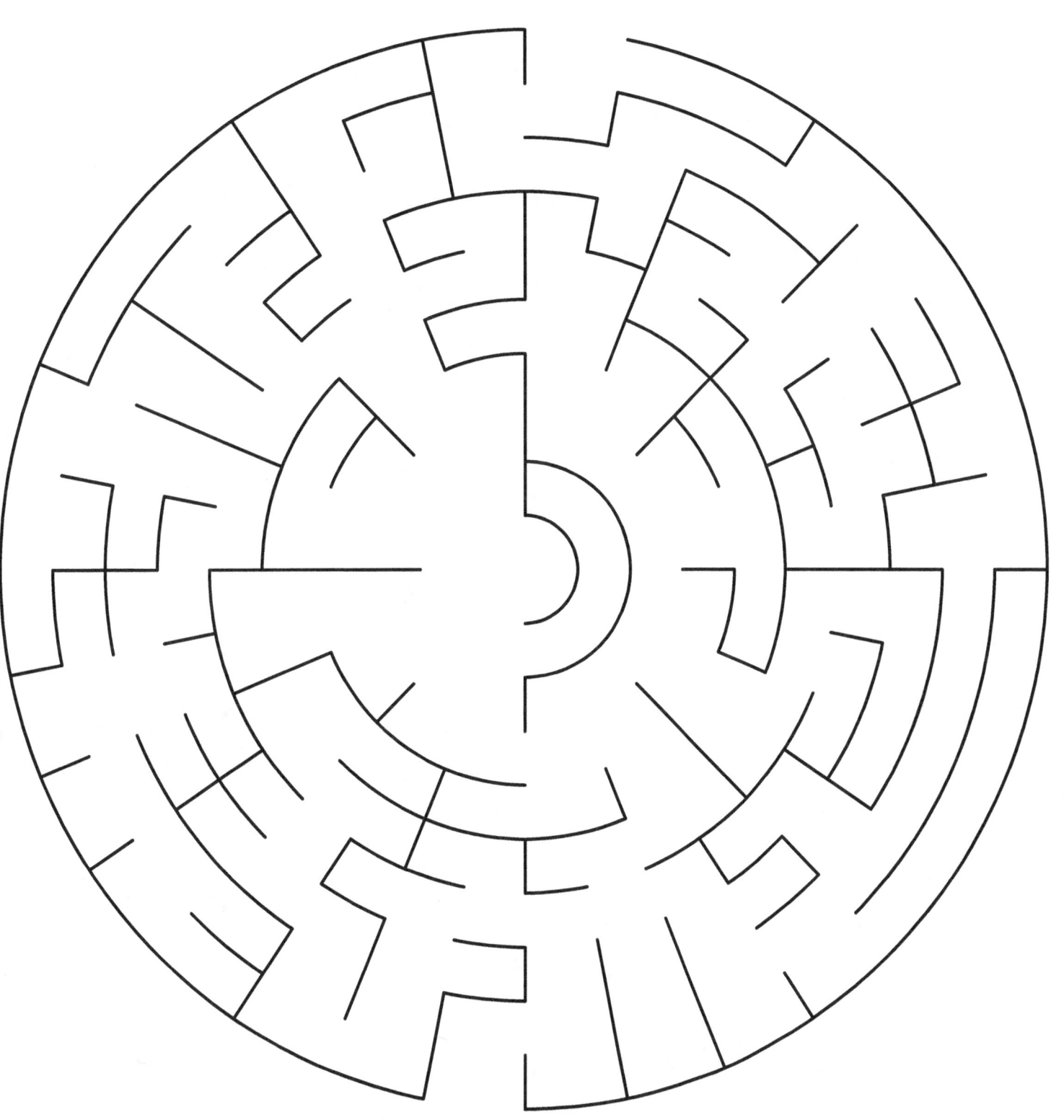

Maze #10

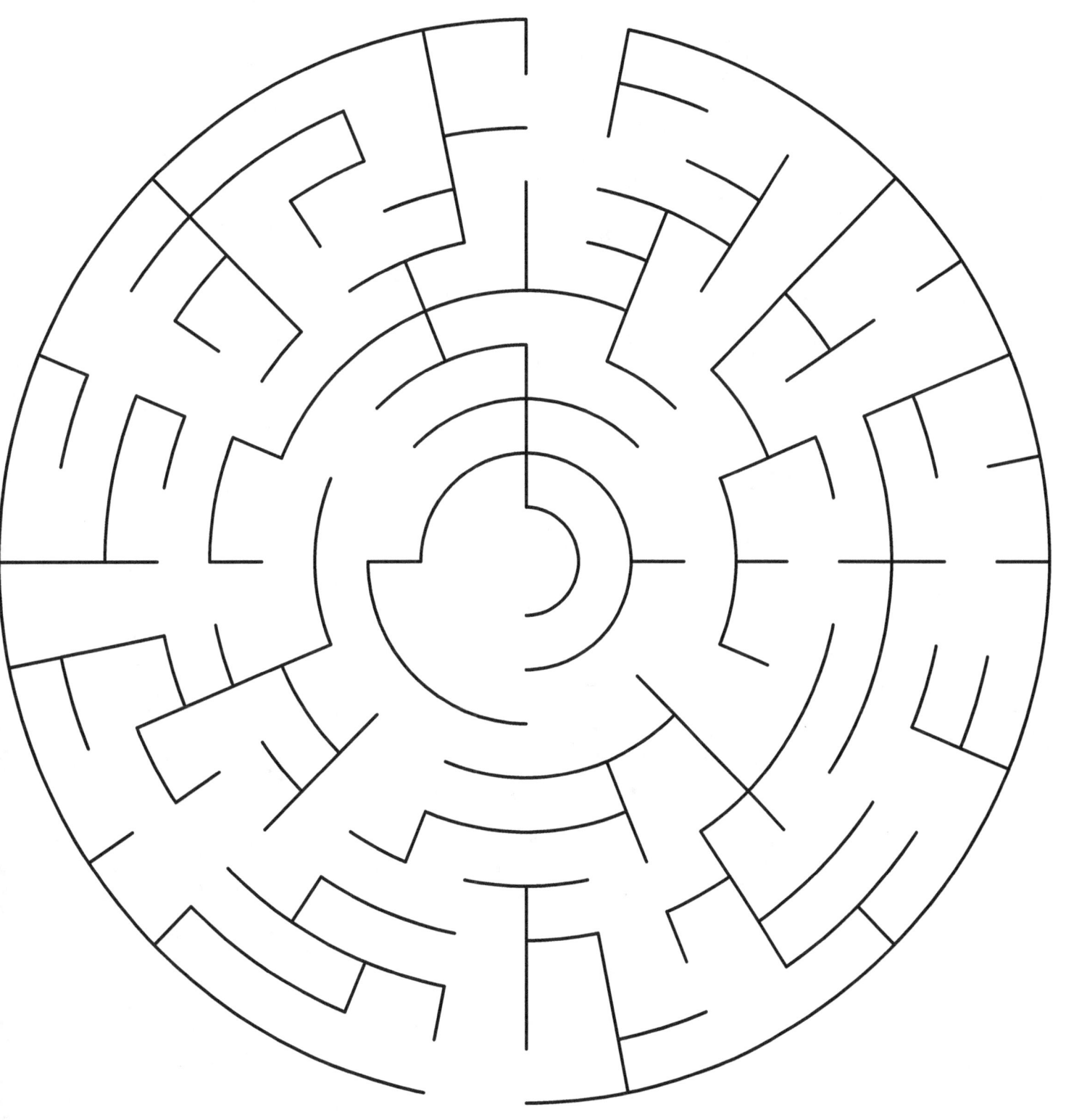

Maze #11

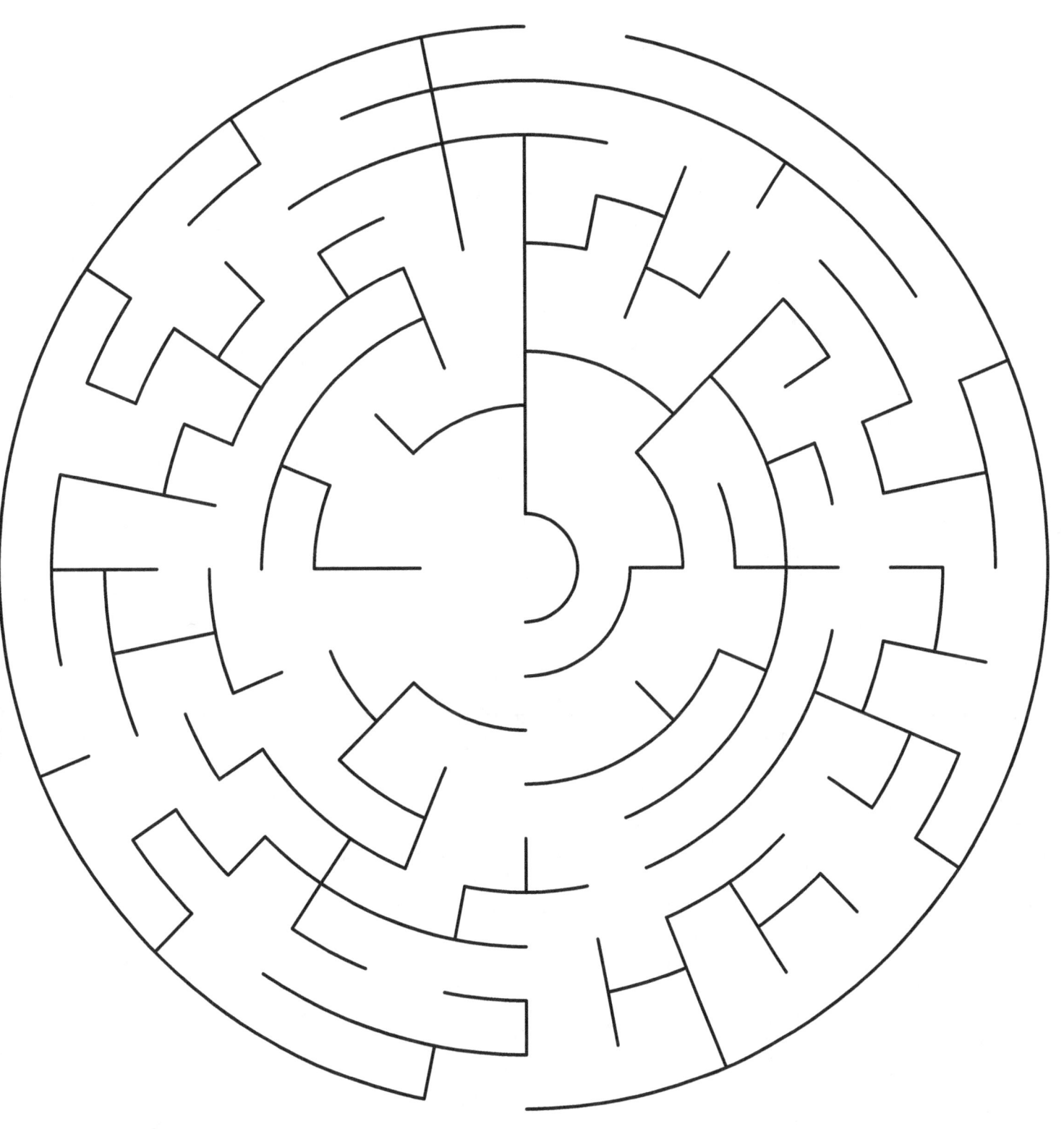

Maze #12

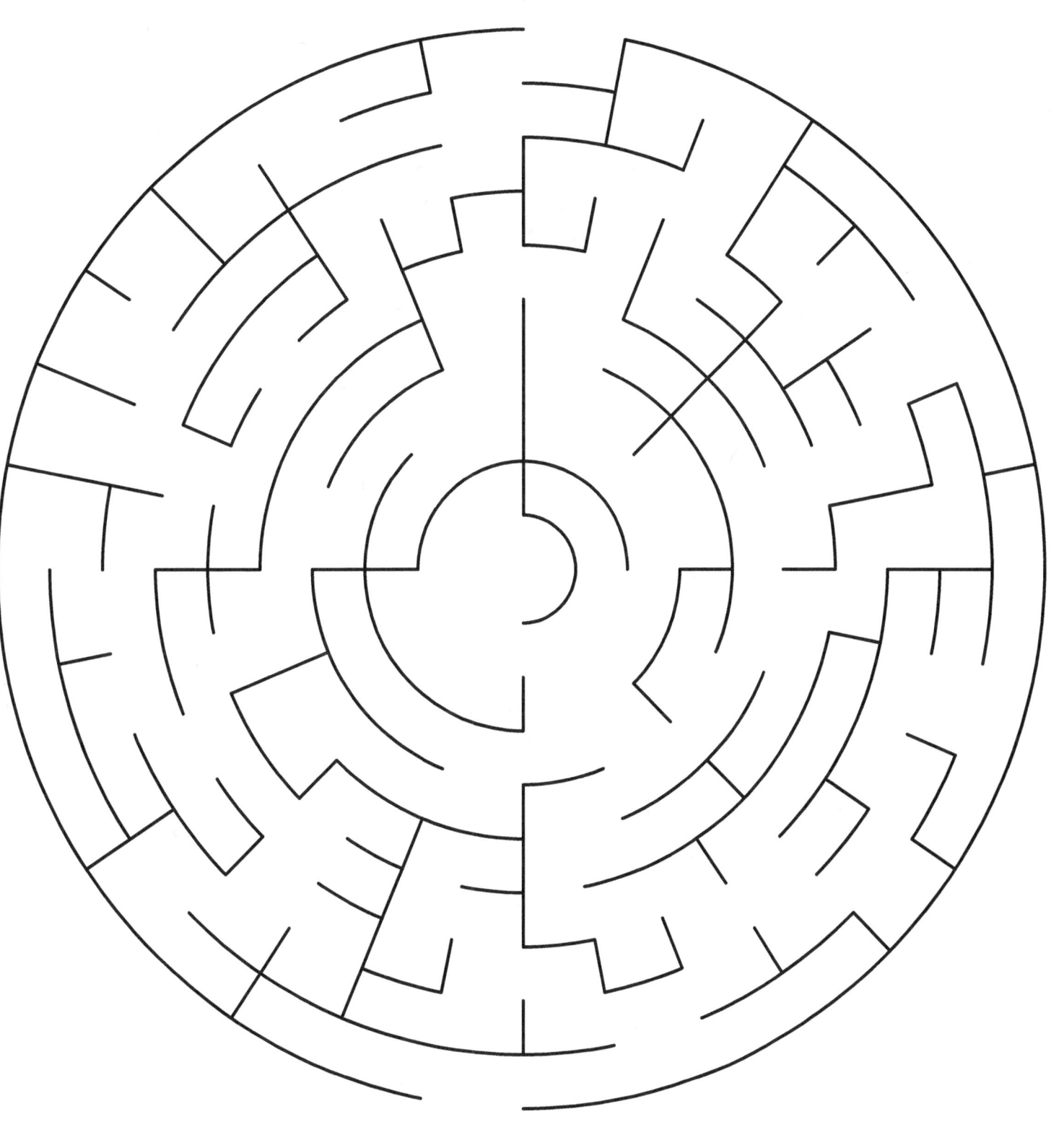

Maze #13

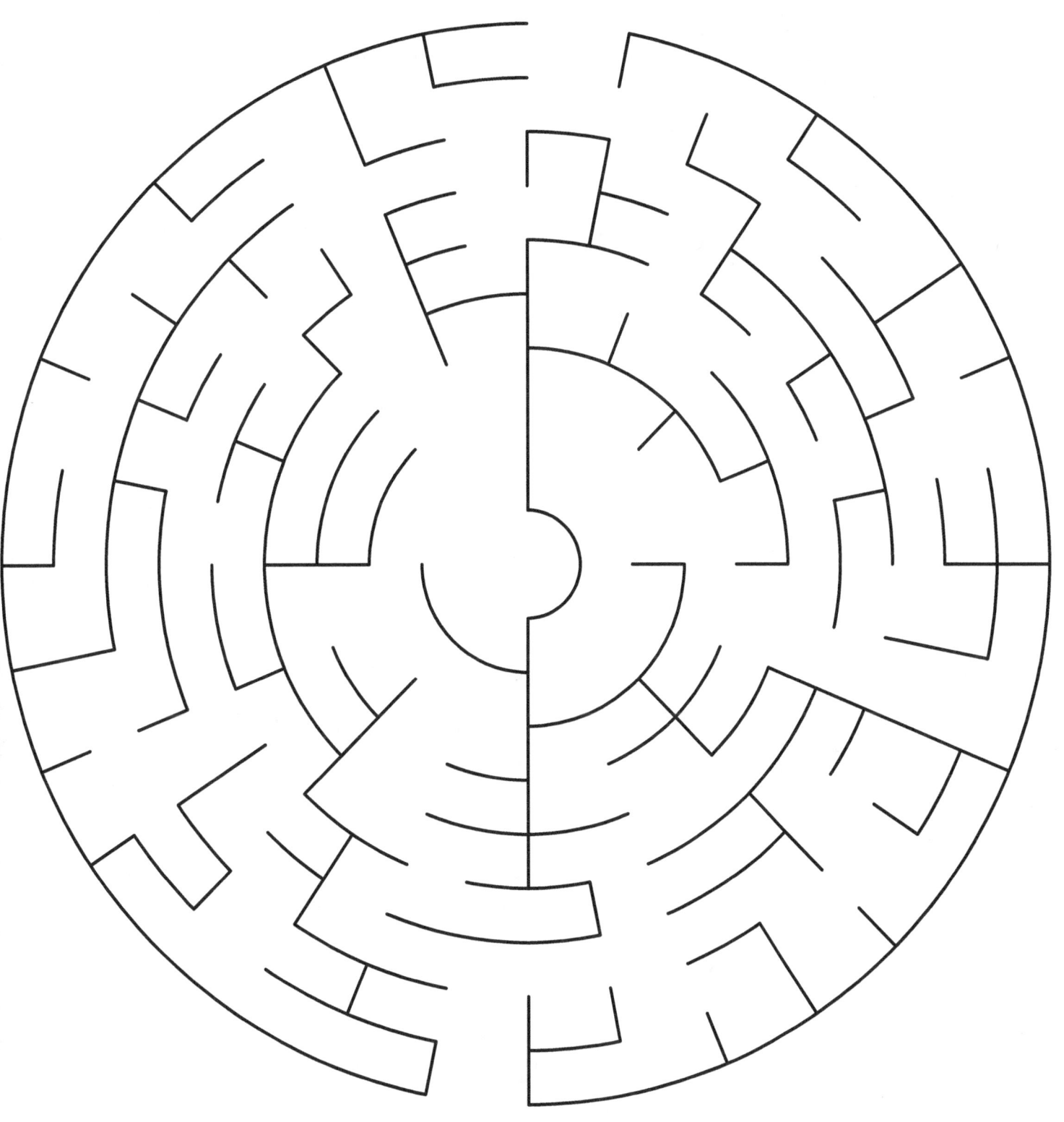

Maze #14

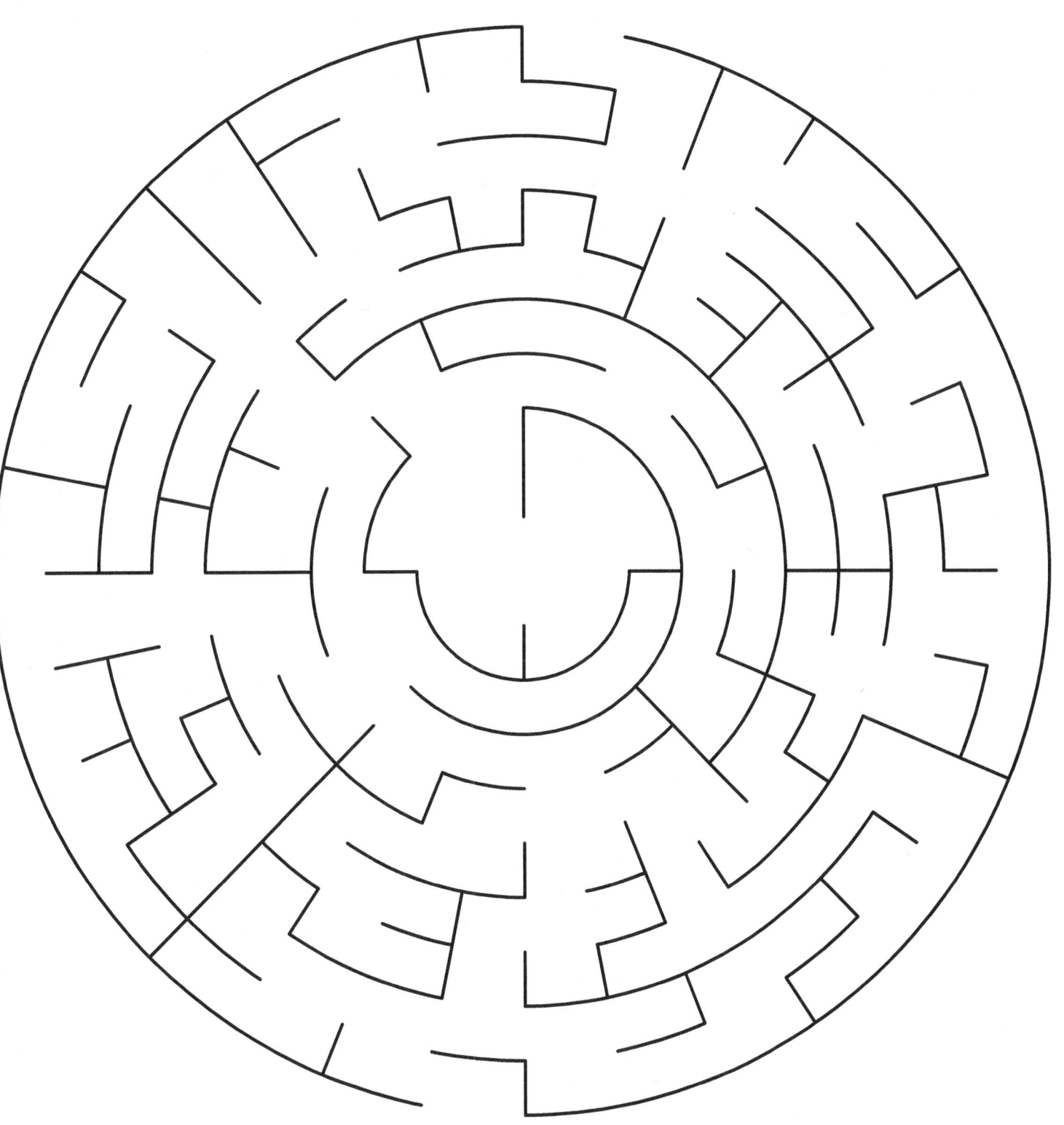

Maze #15

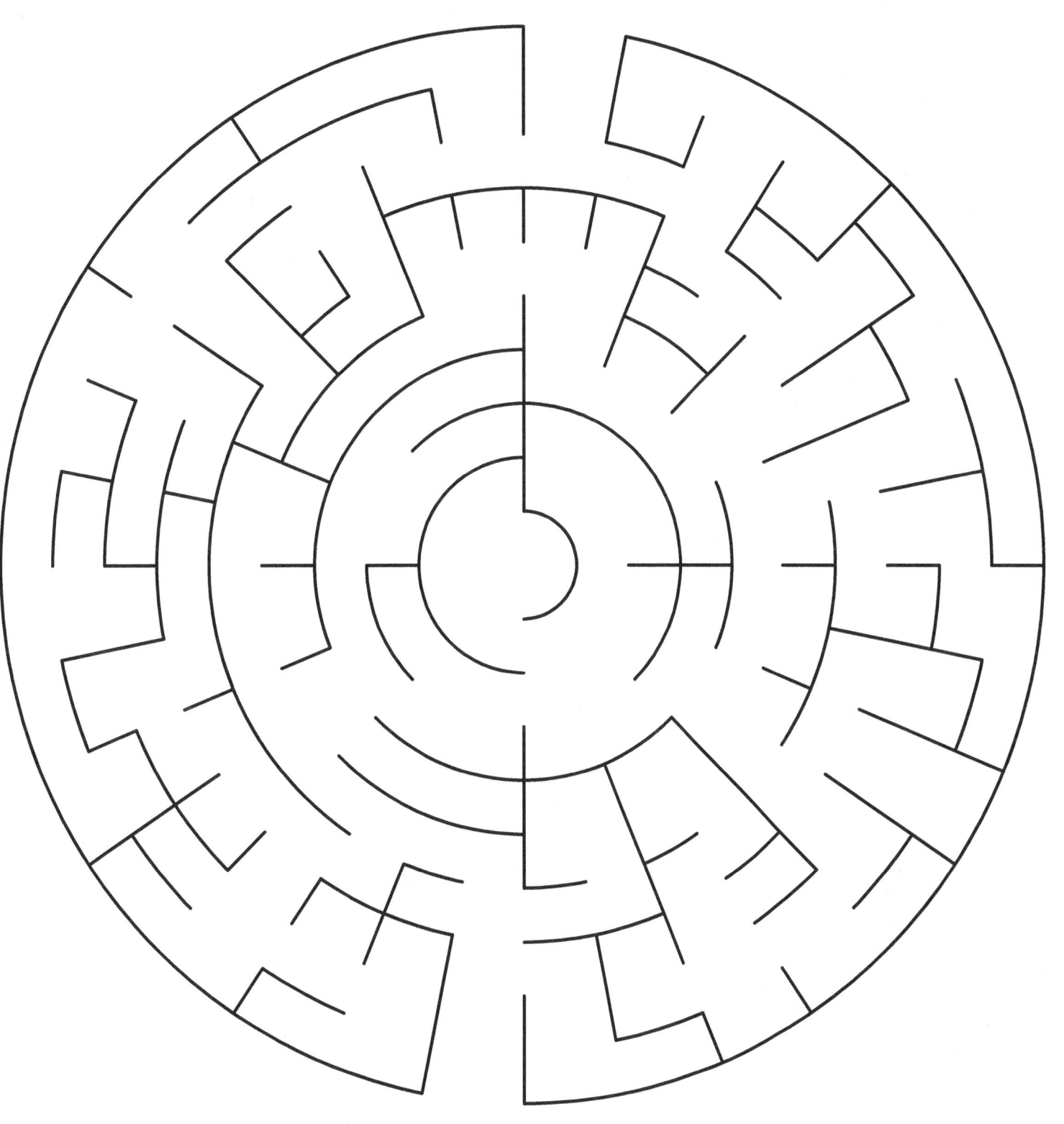

Maze #16

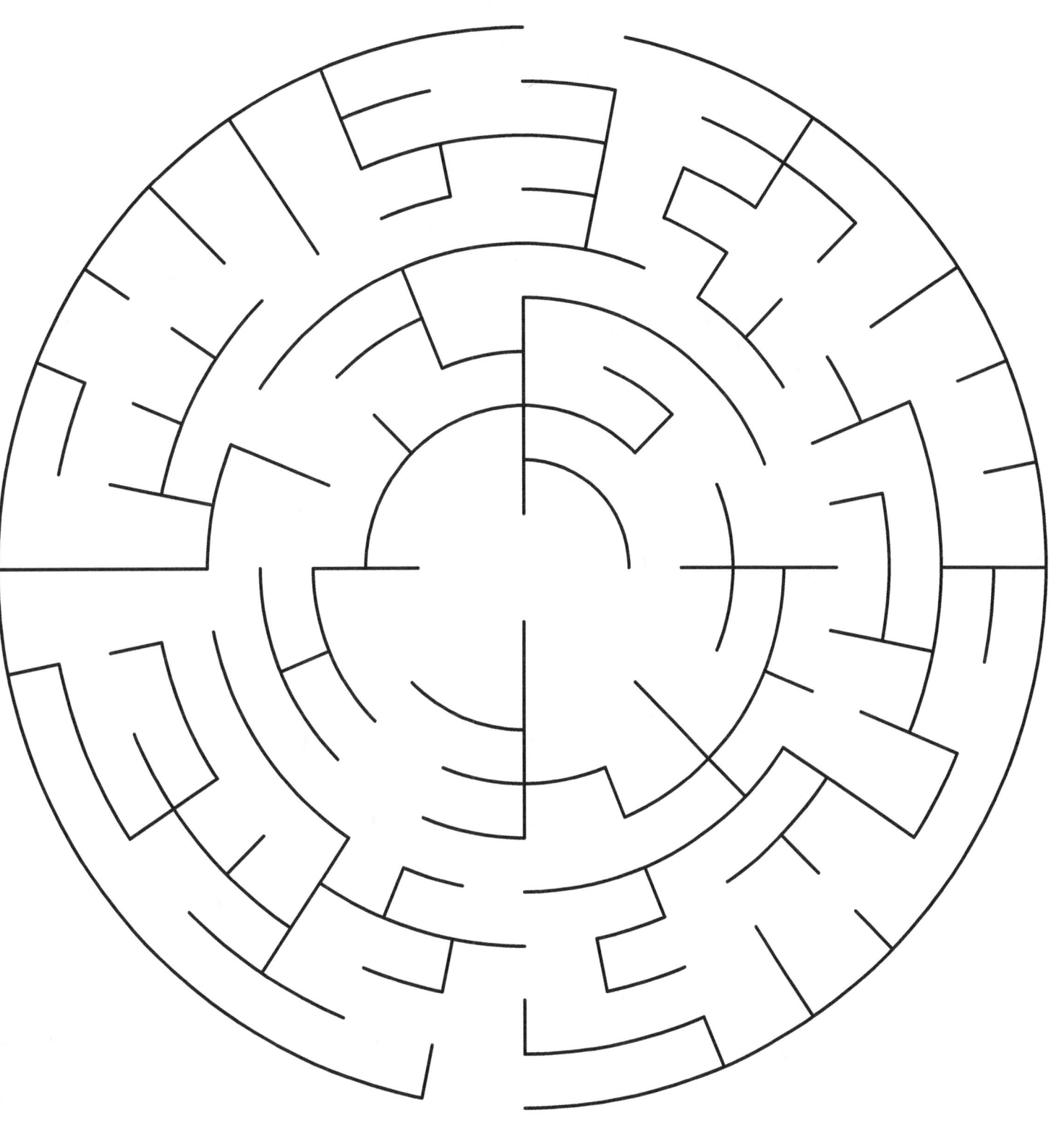

Maze #17

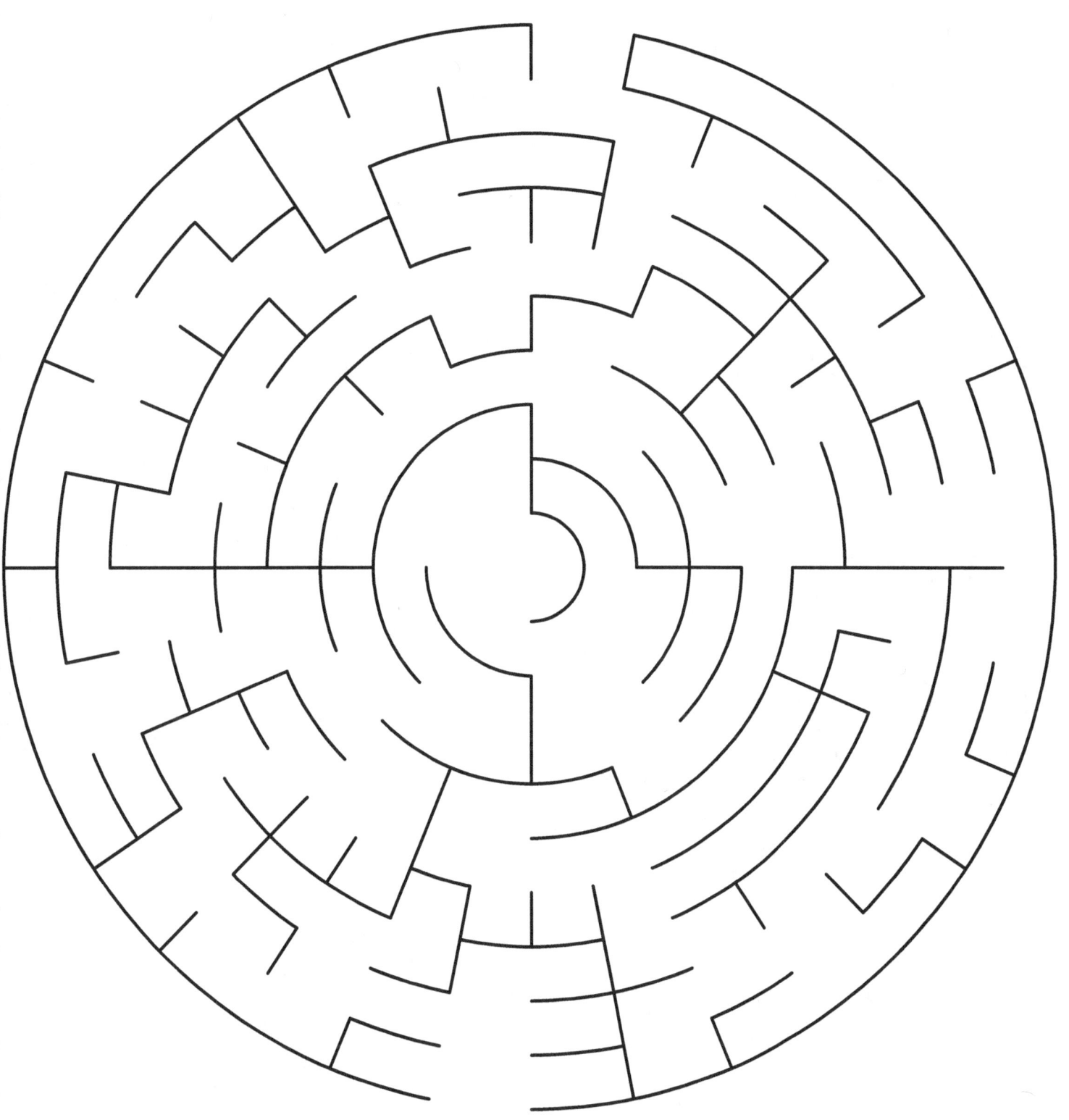

Maze #18

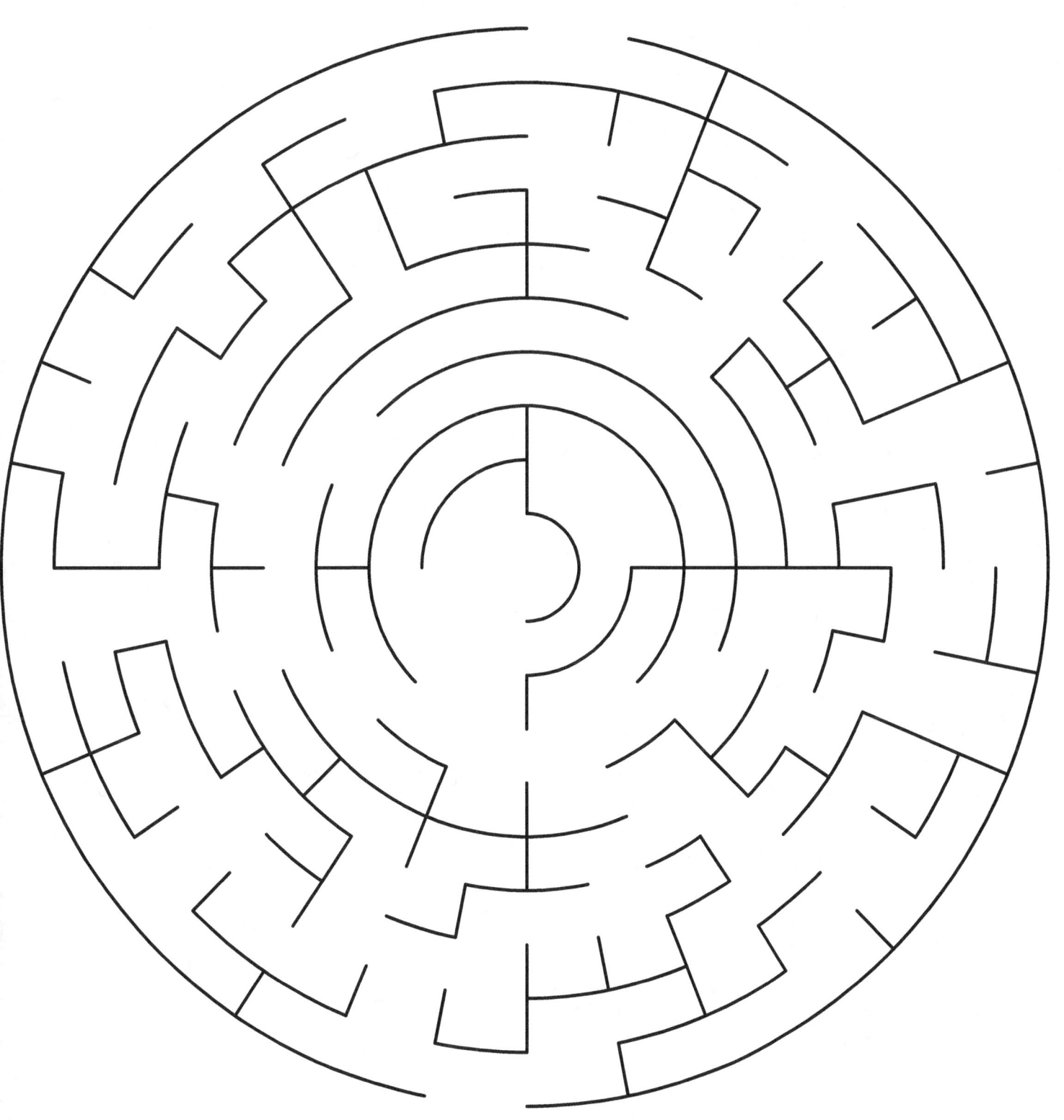

Maze #19

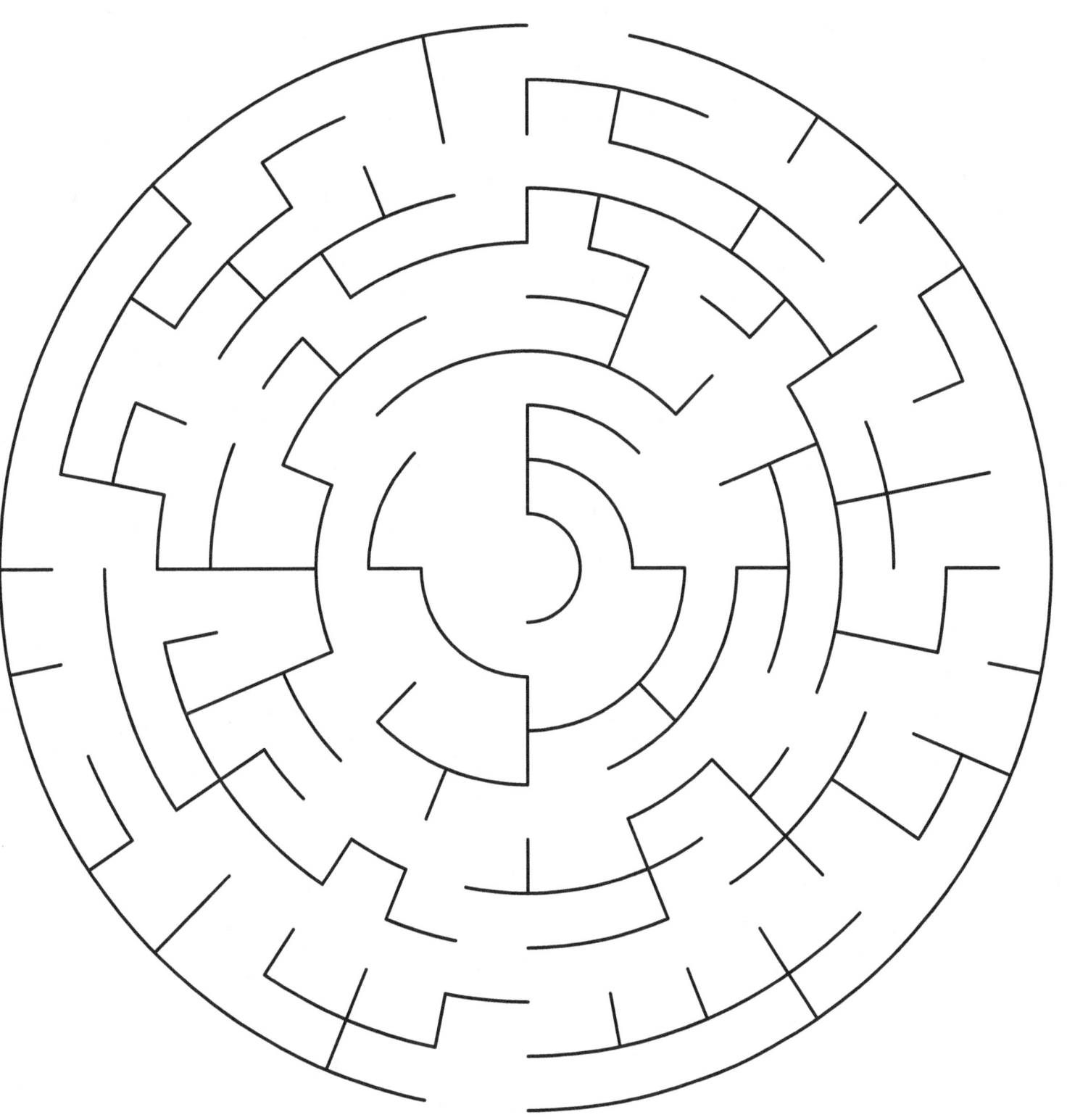

Maze #20

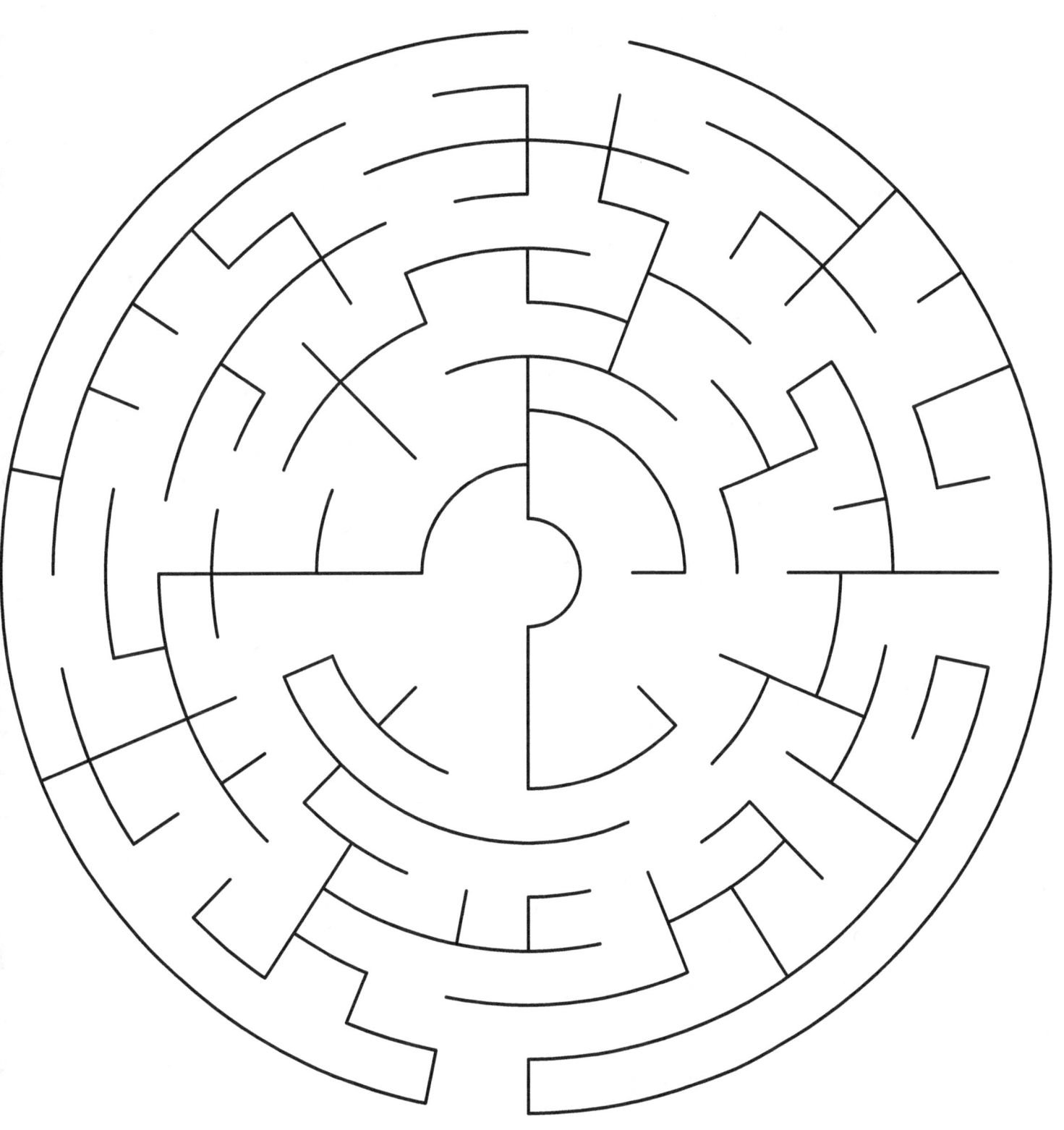

Maze #21

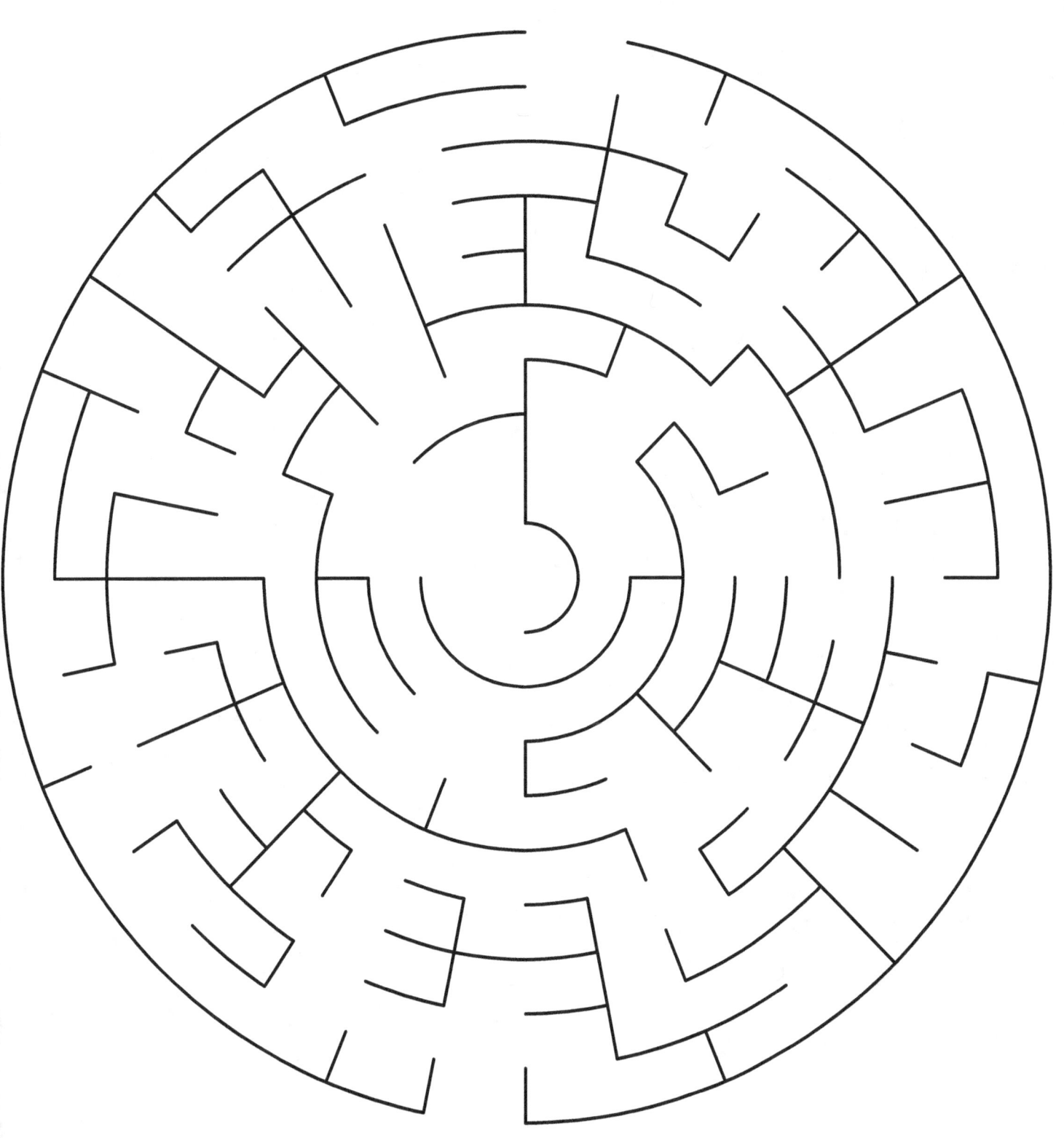

Maze #22

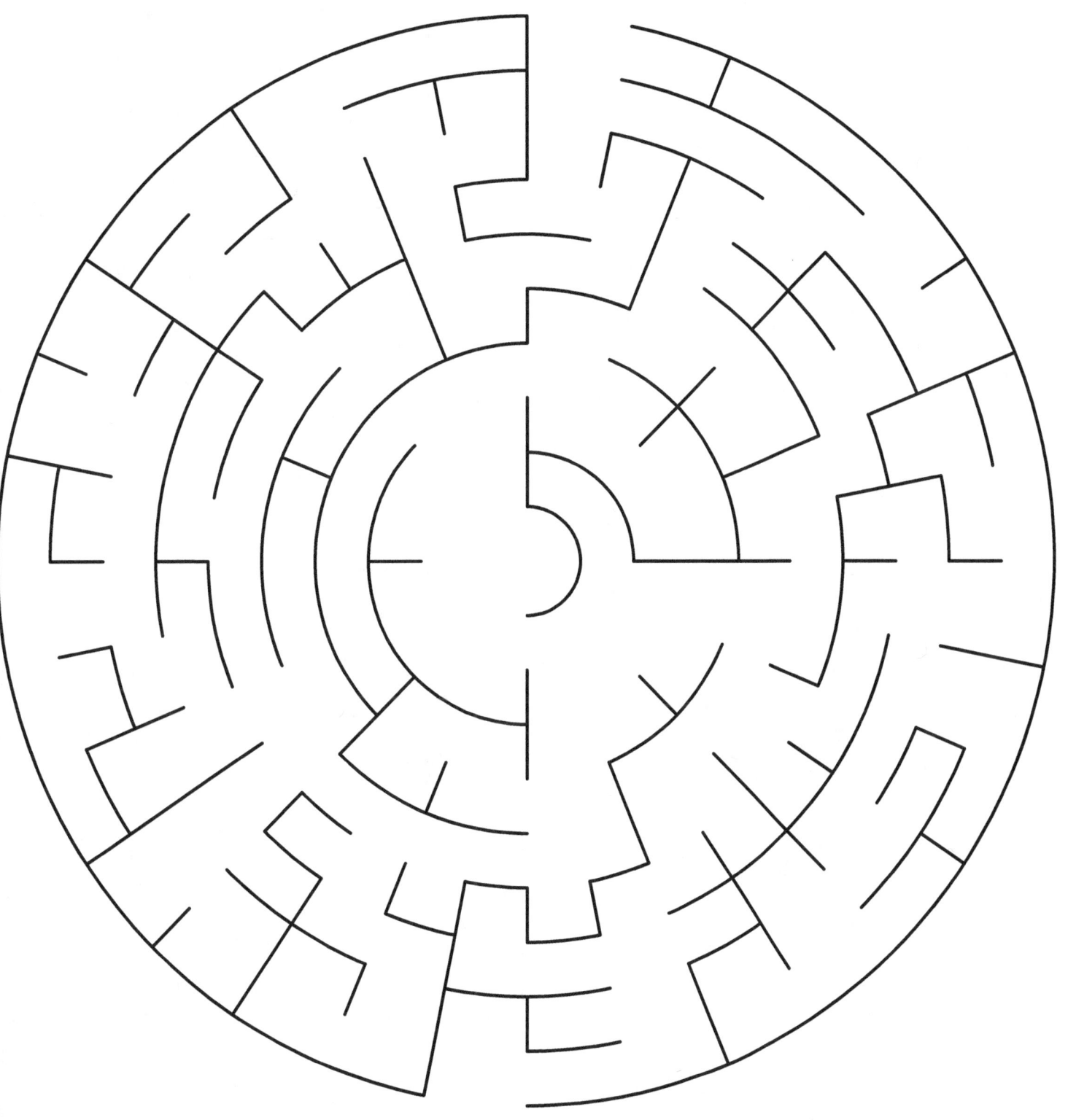

Maze #23

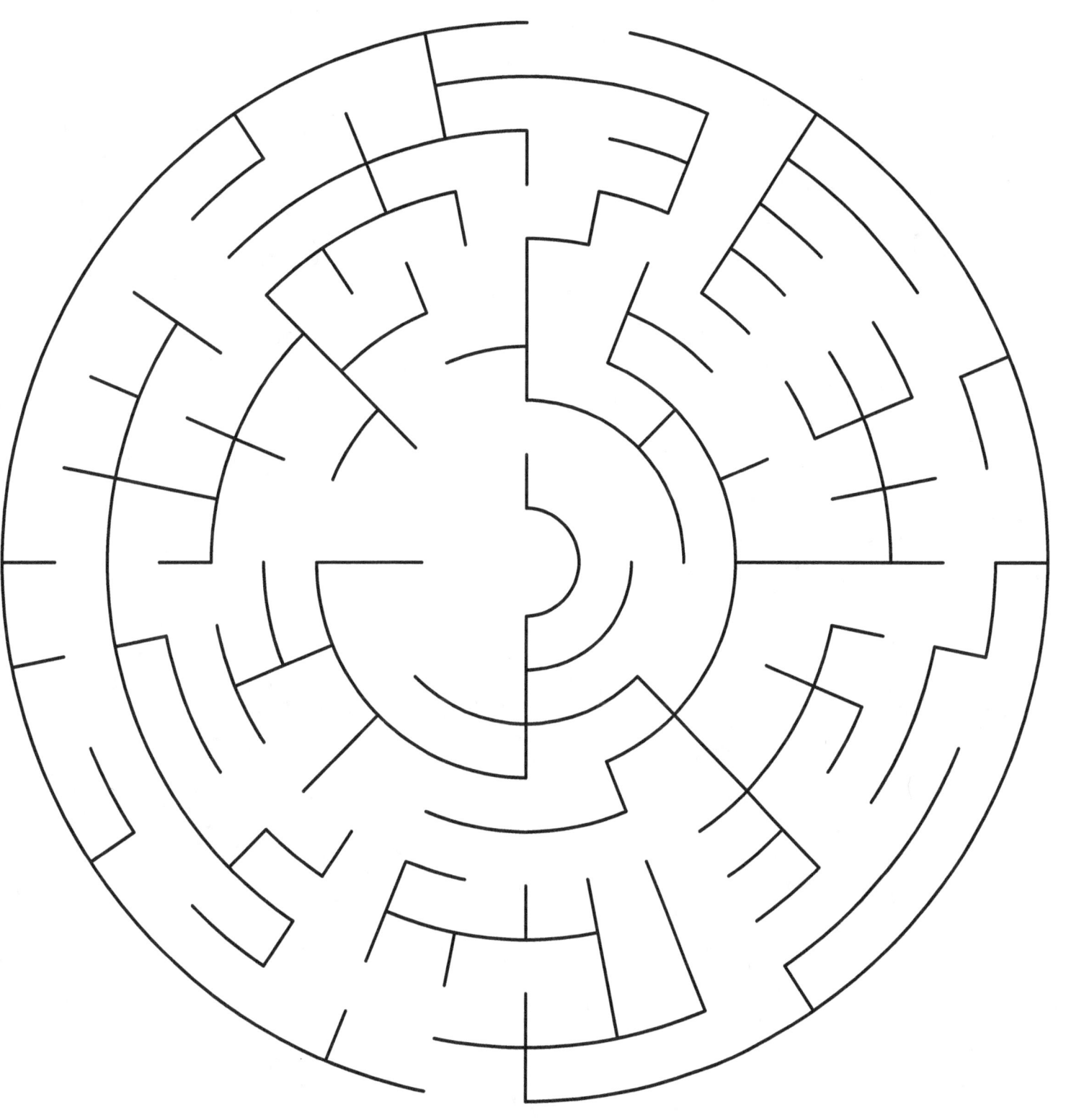

Maze #24

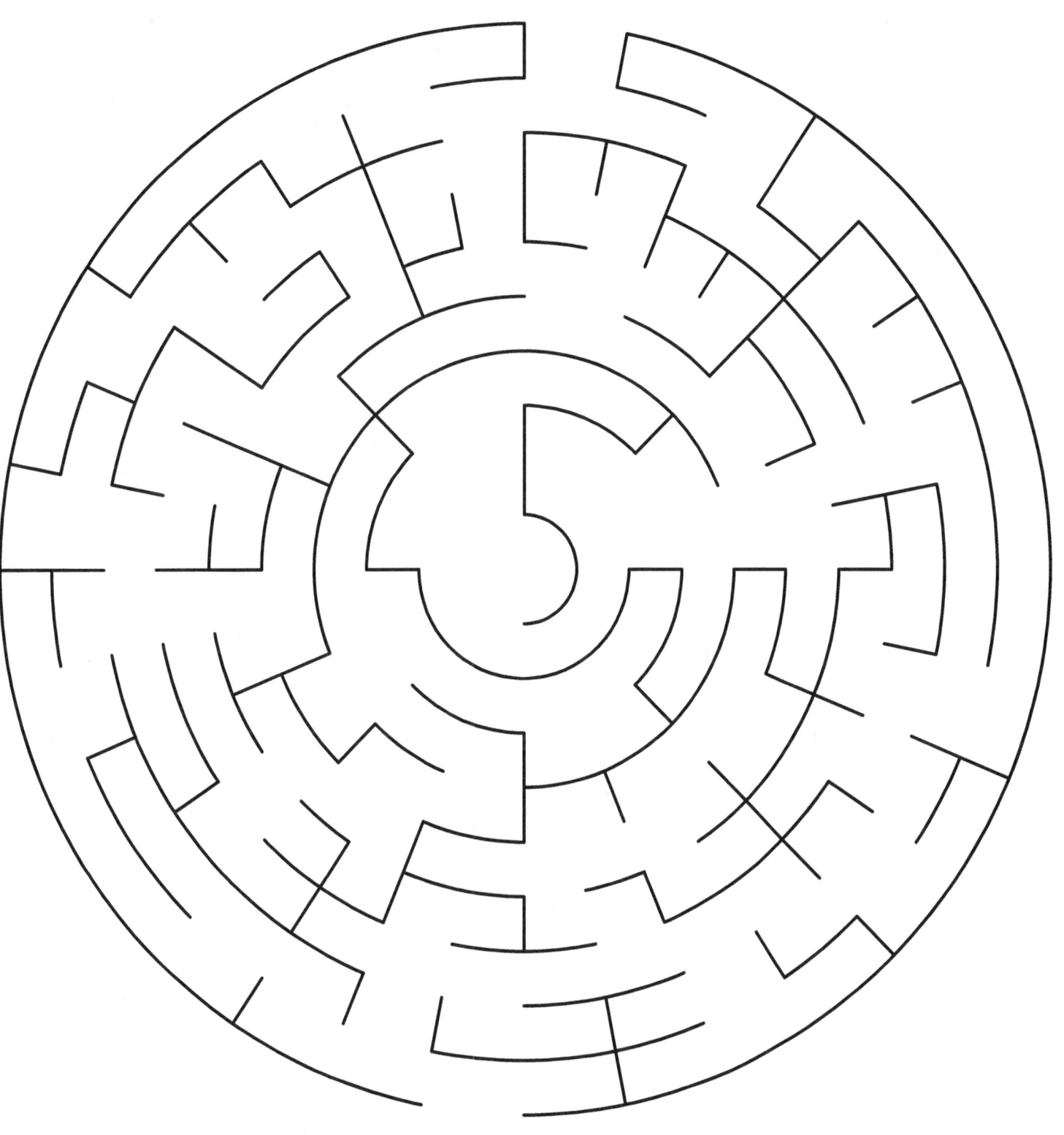

Maze #25

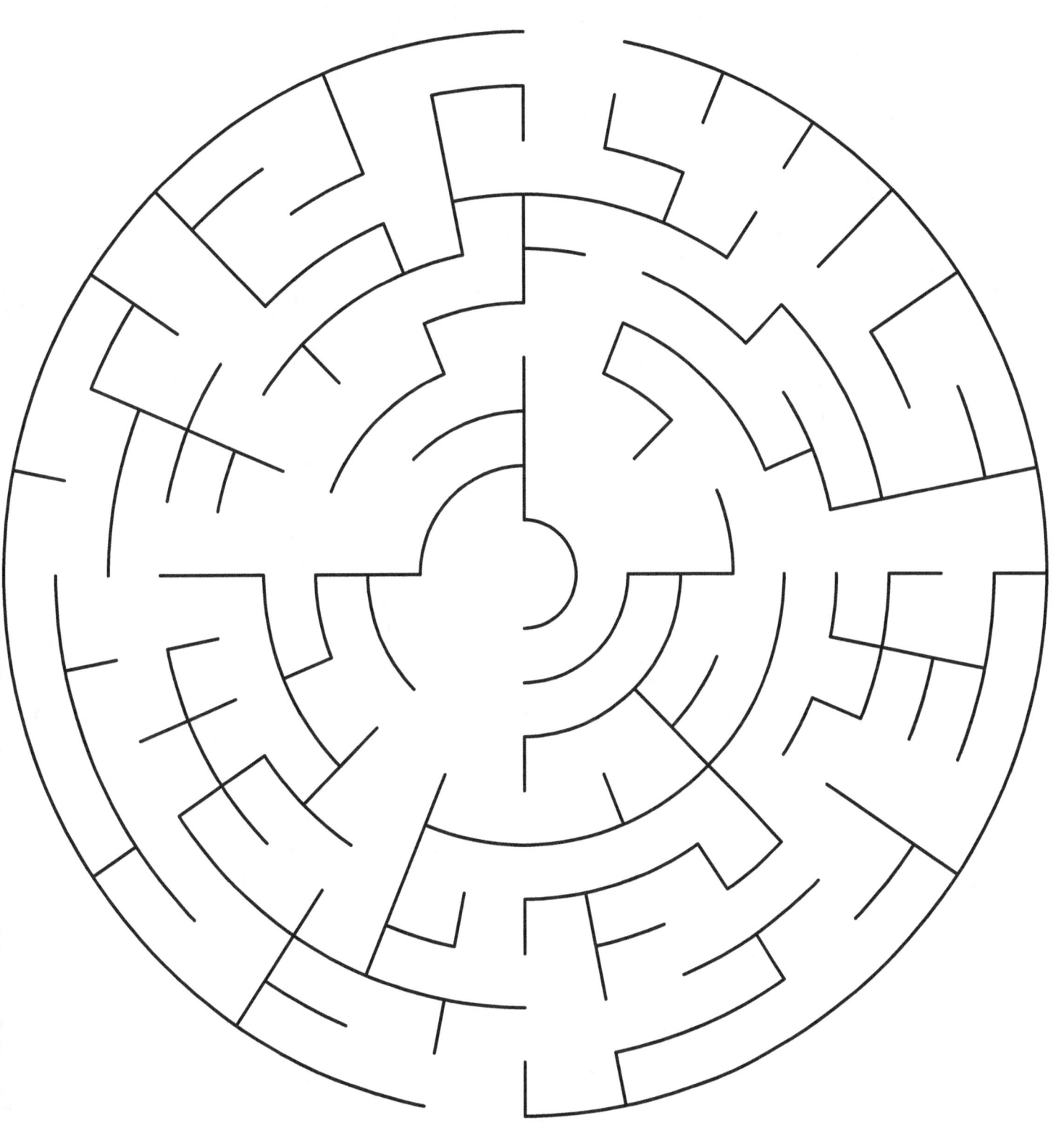

Maze #26

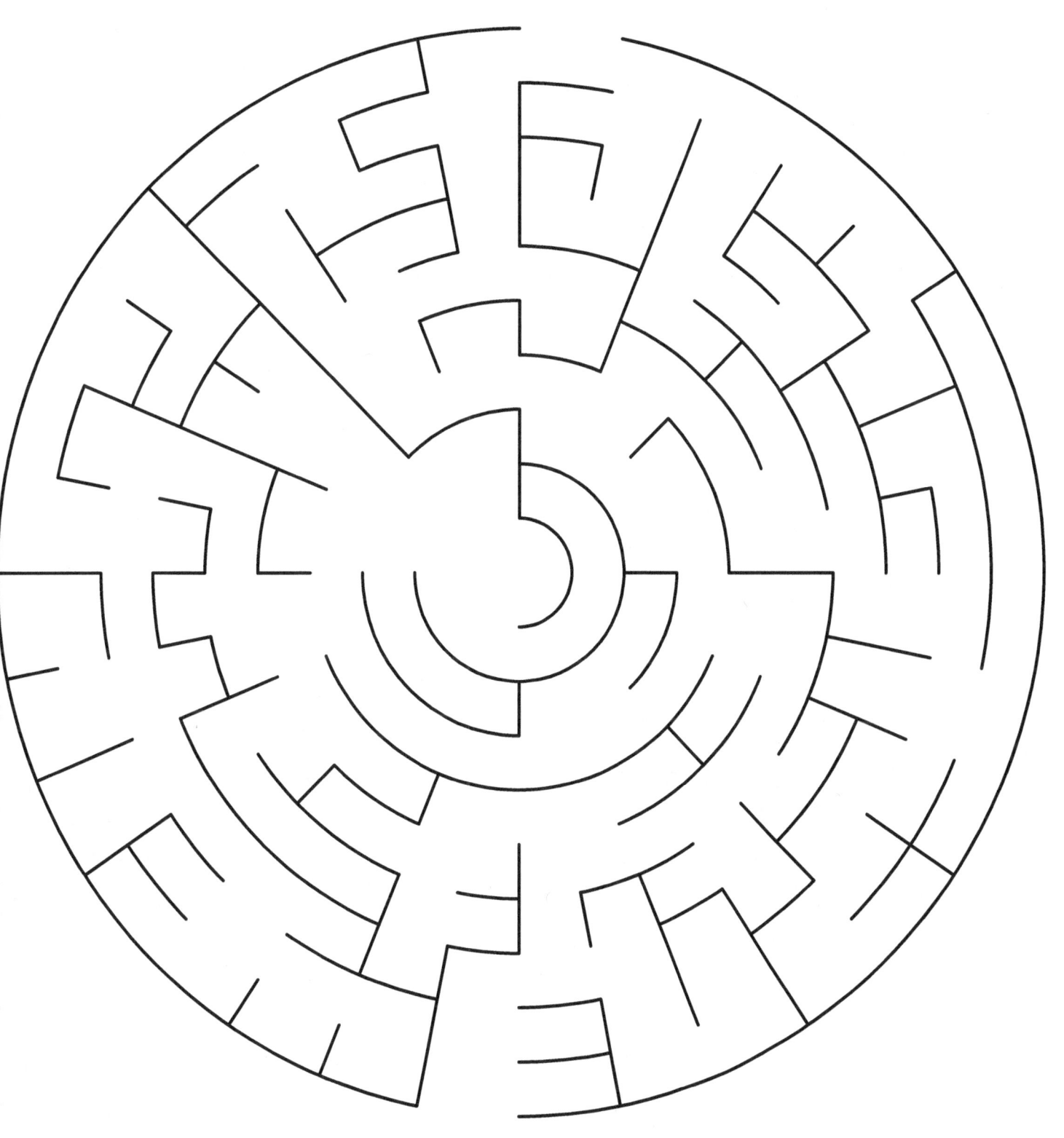

Maze #27

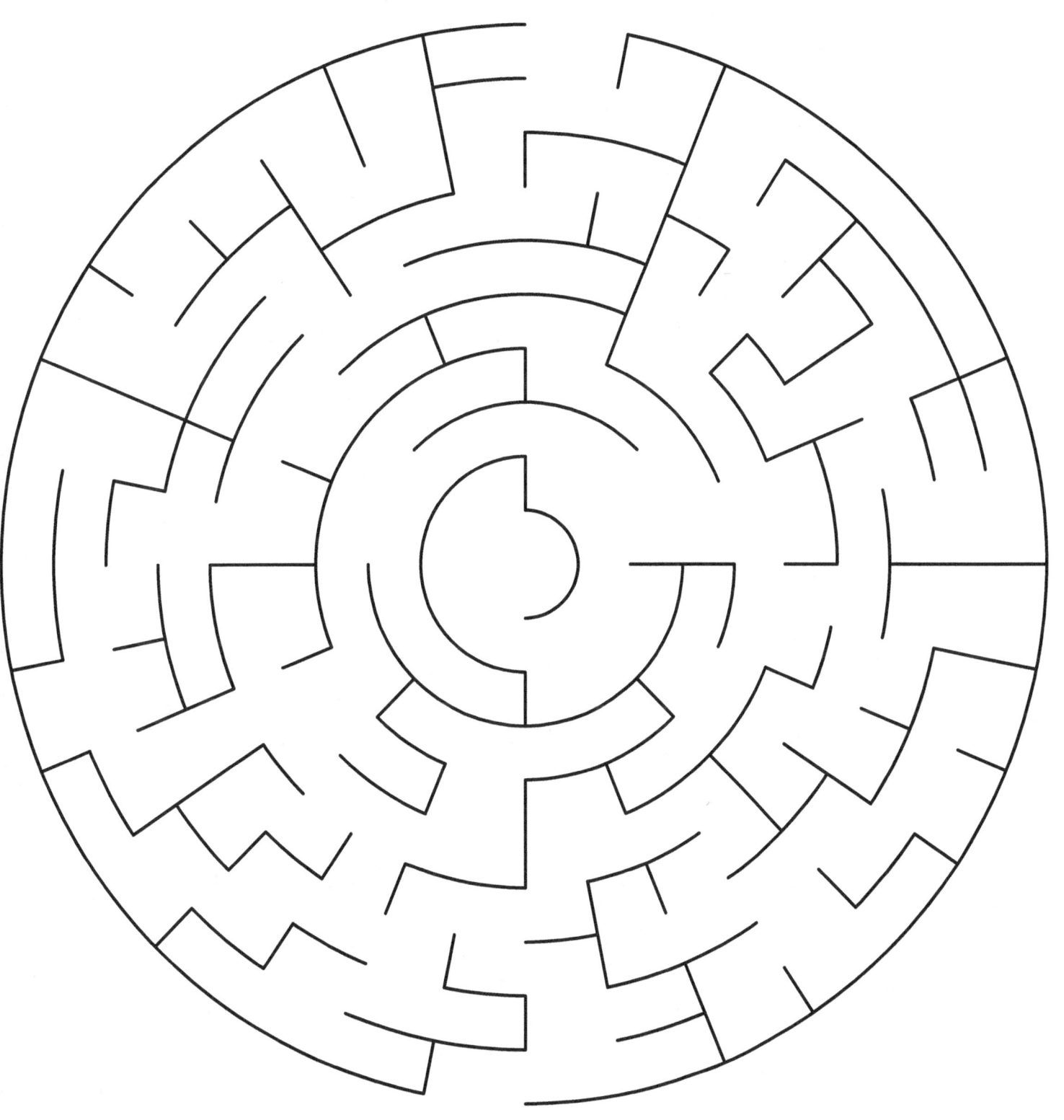

Maze #28

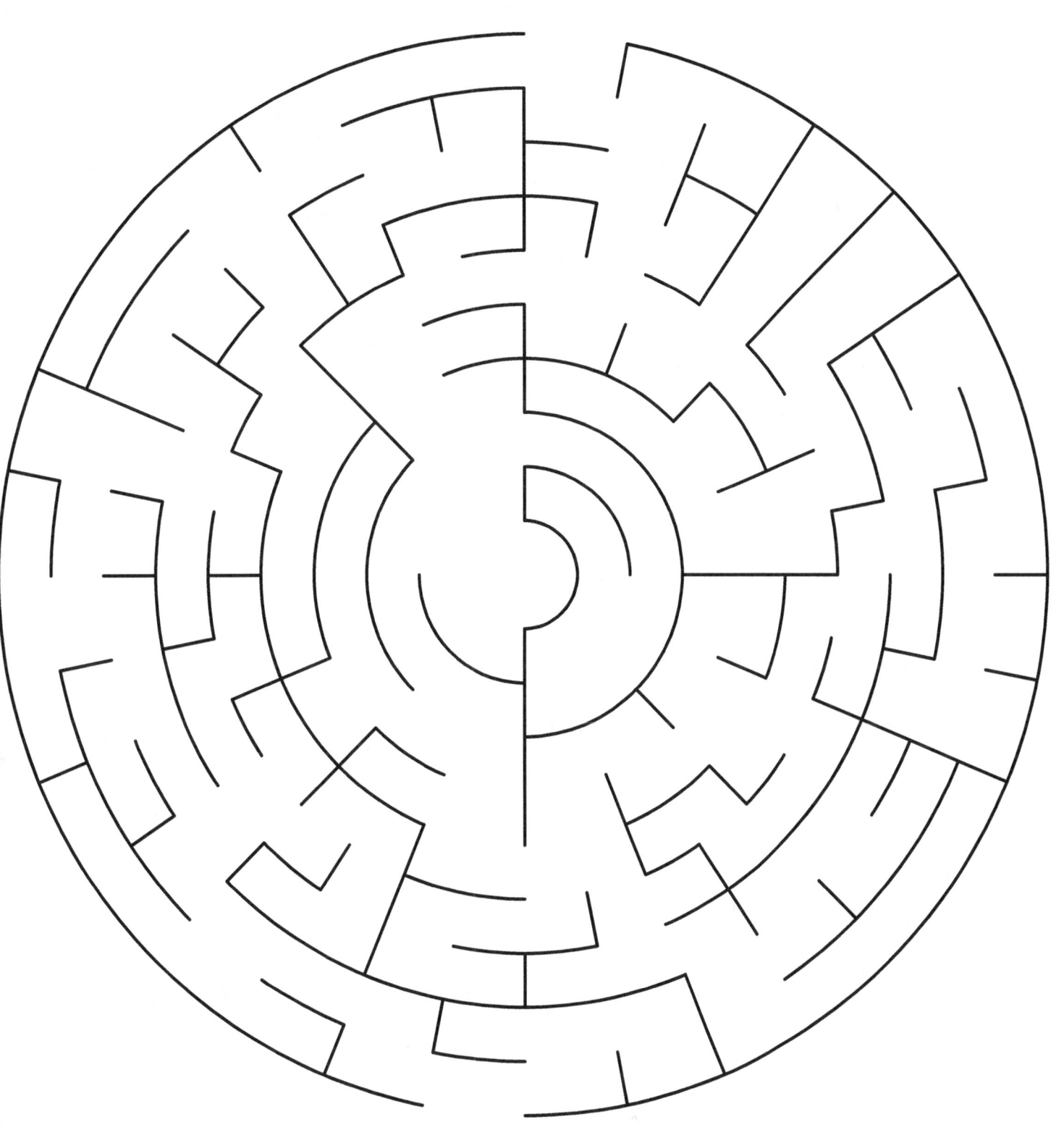

Maze #29

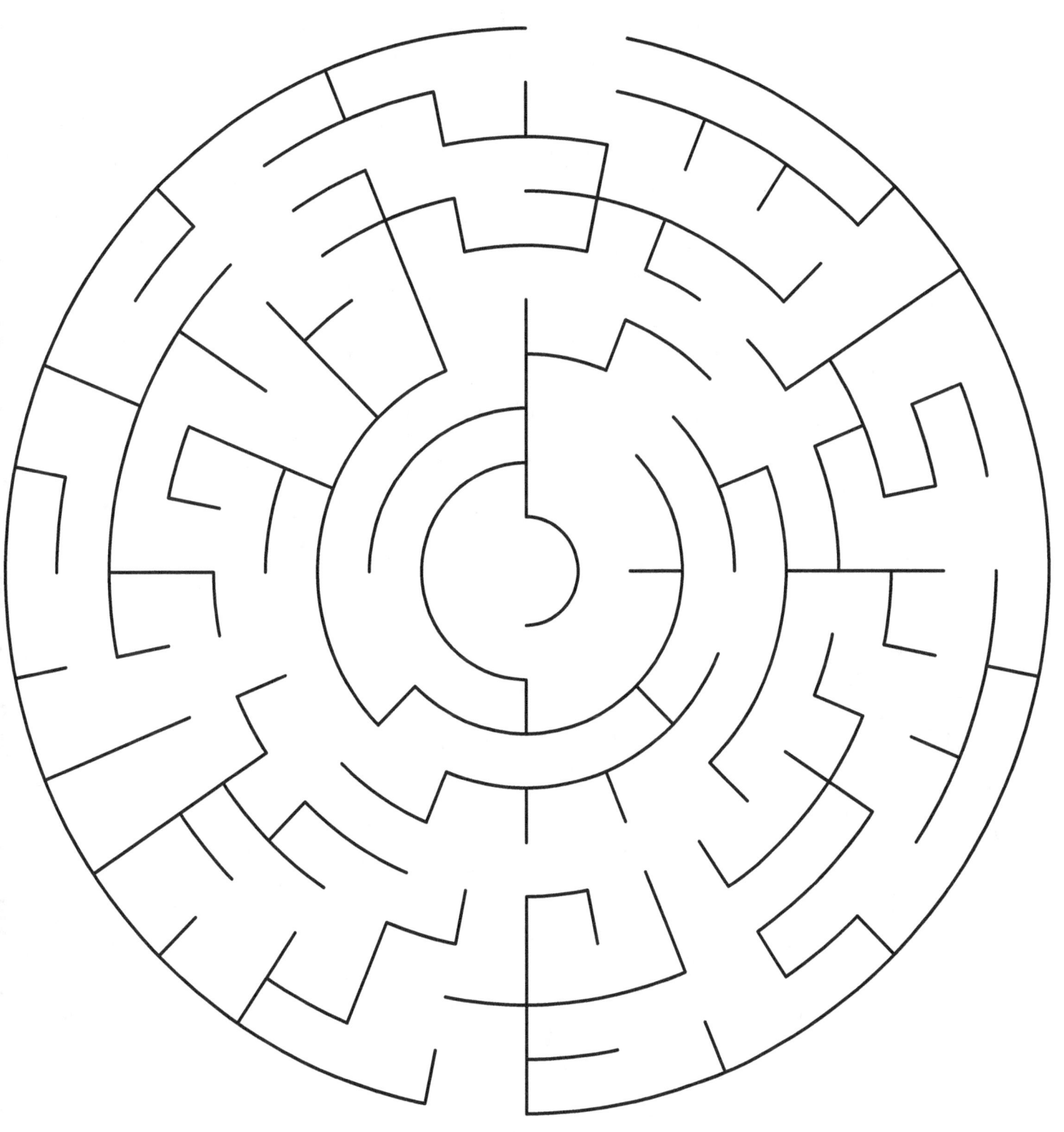

Maze #30

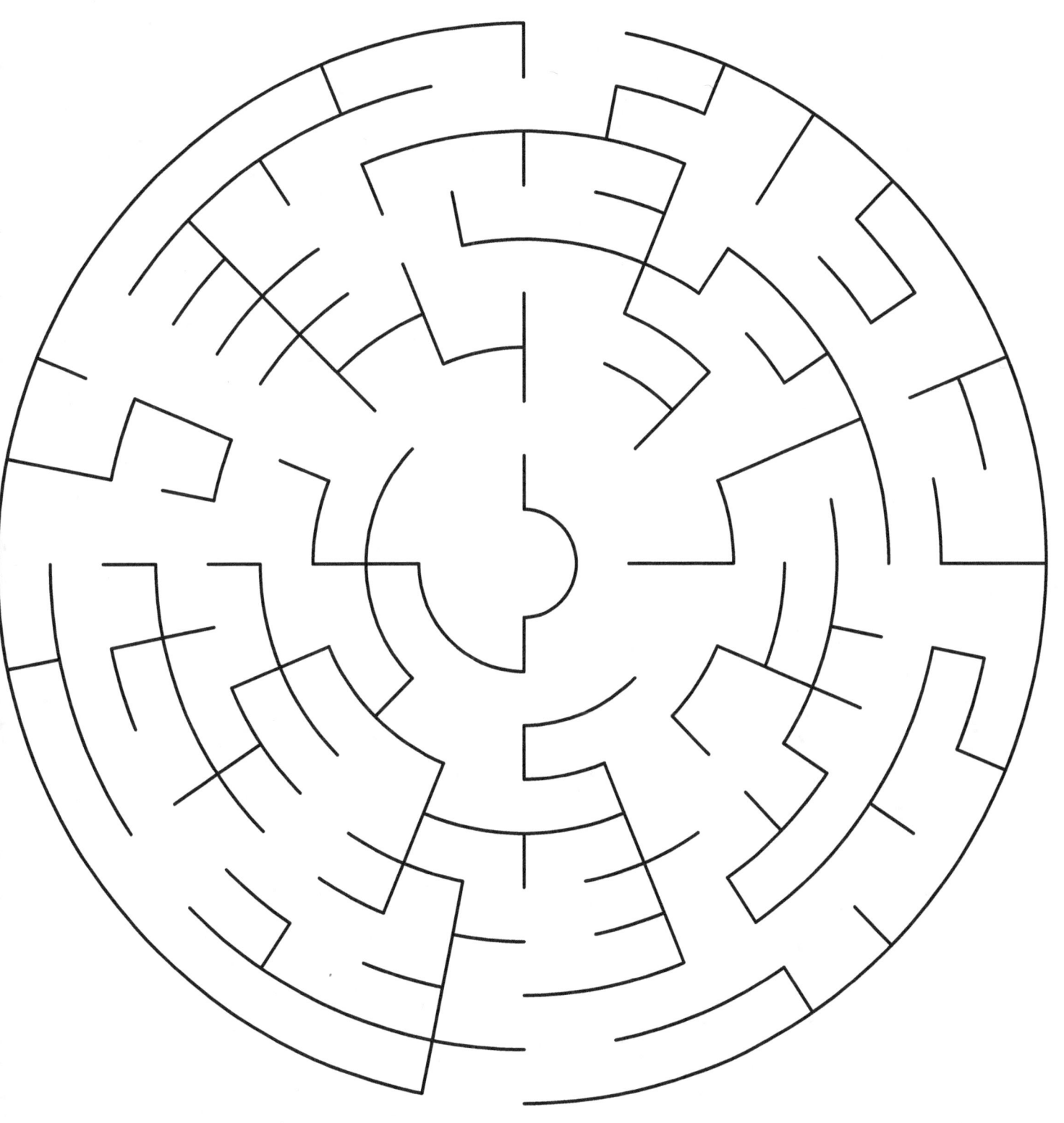

Maze #31

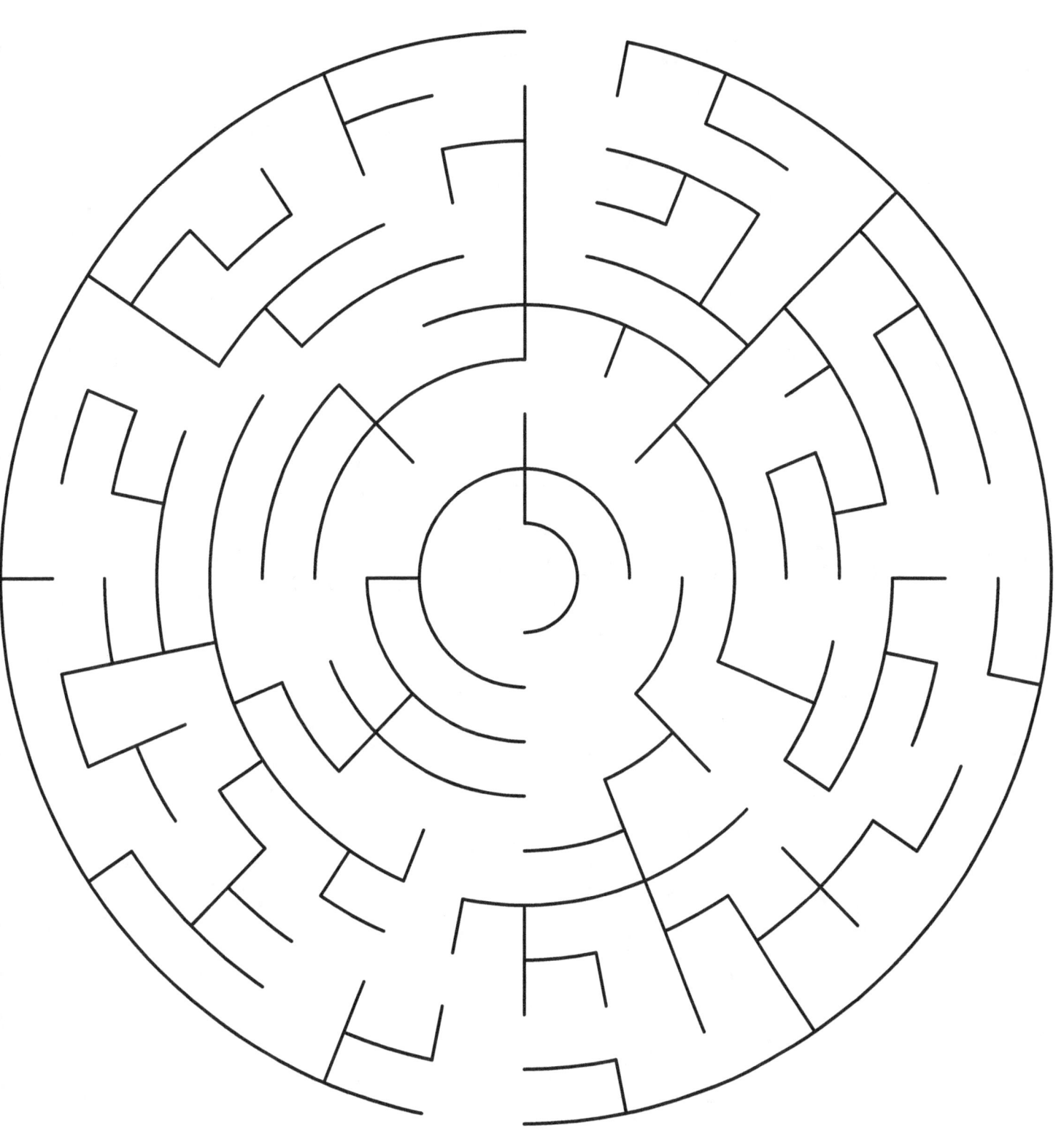

Maze #32

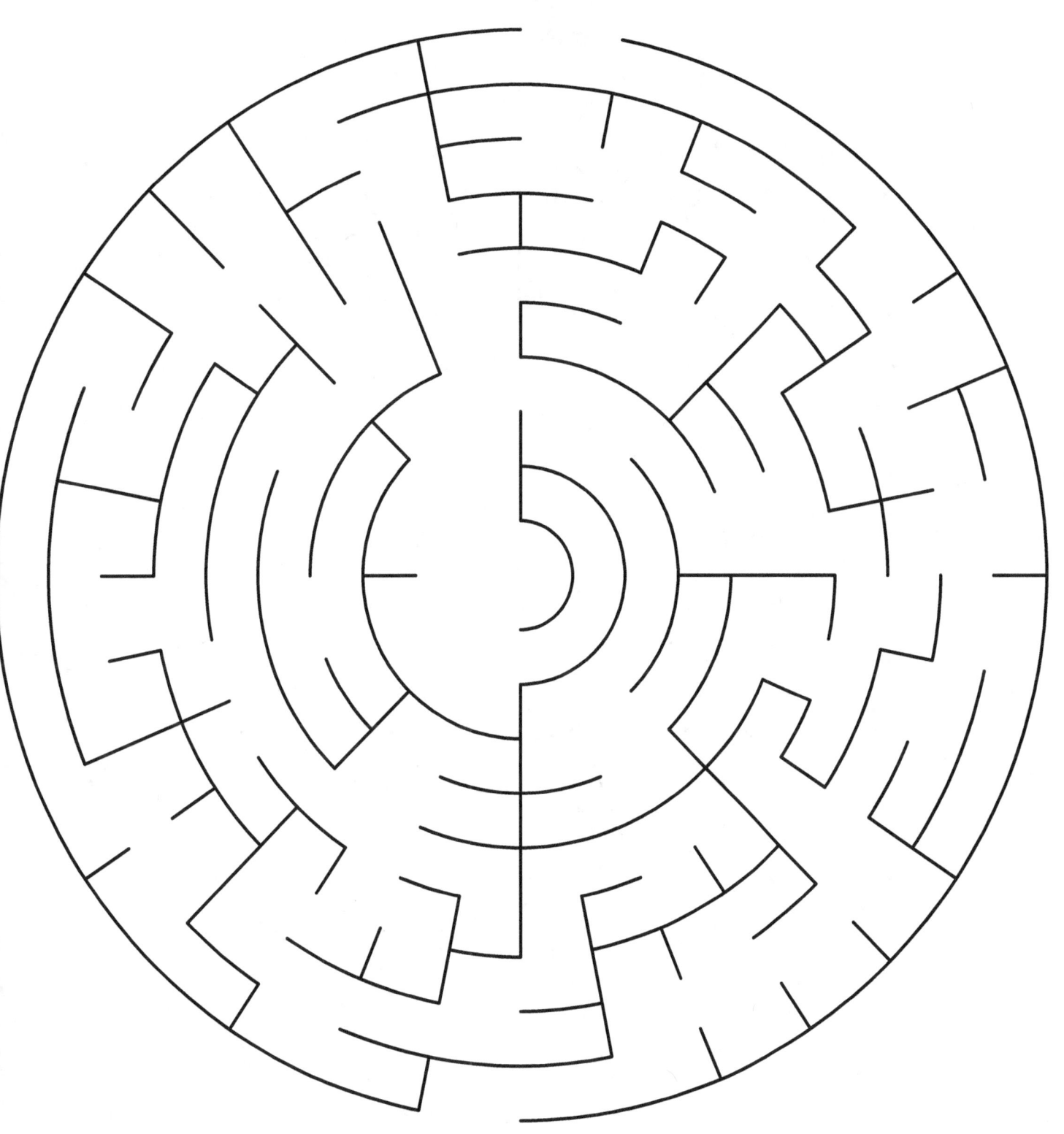

Maze Solution #1

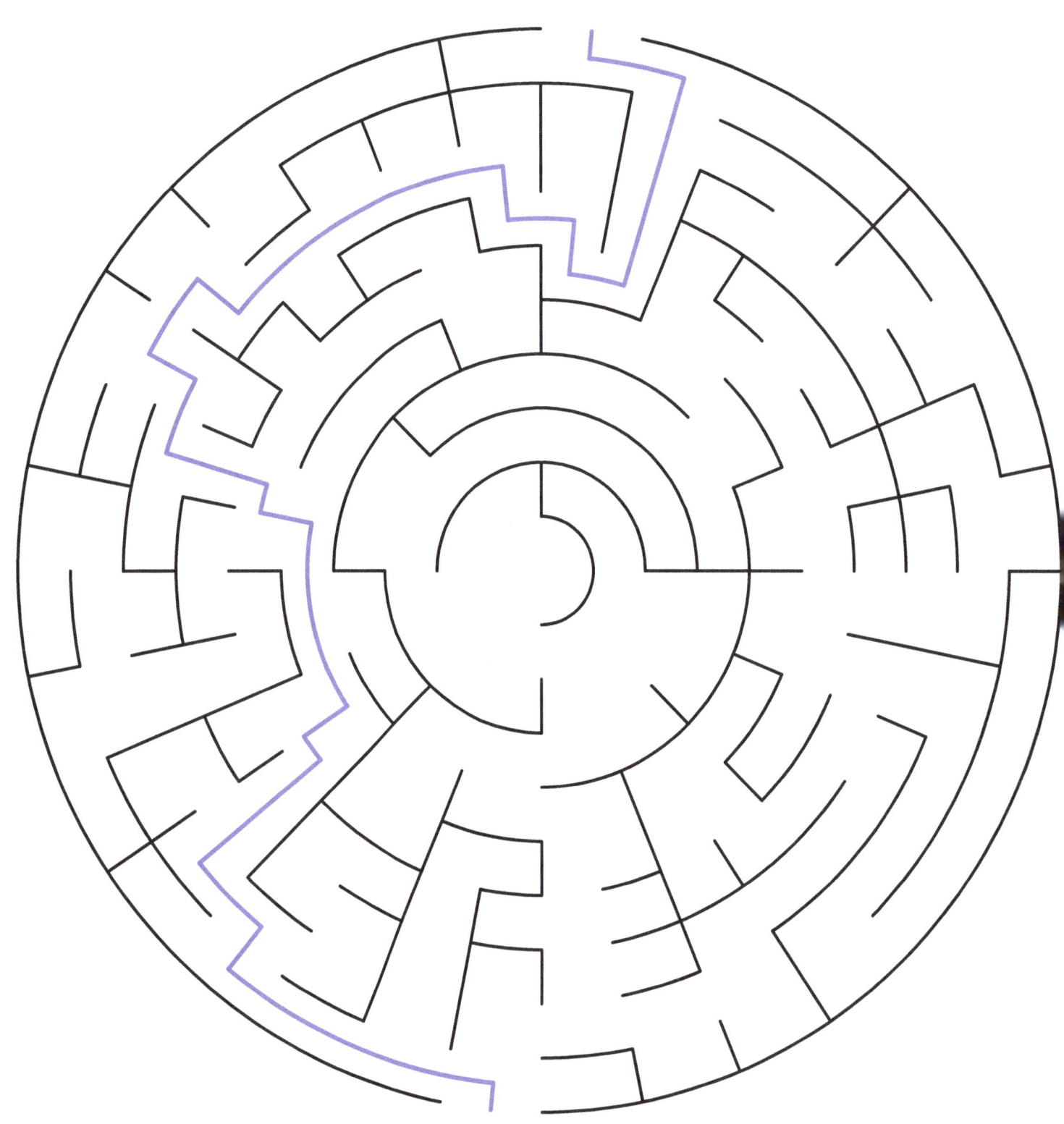

Maze Solution #2

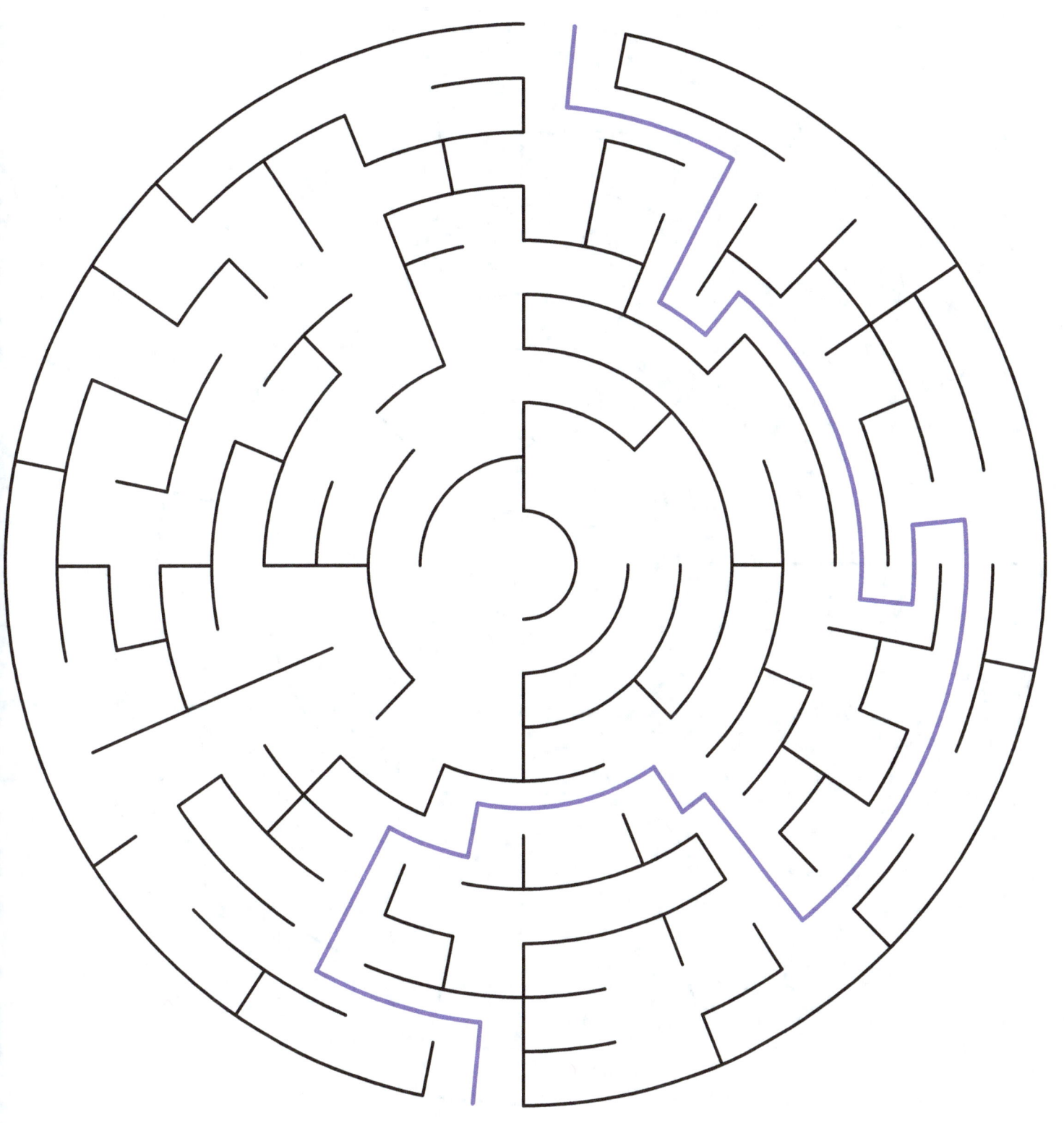

Maze Solution #3

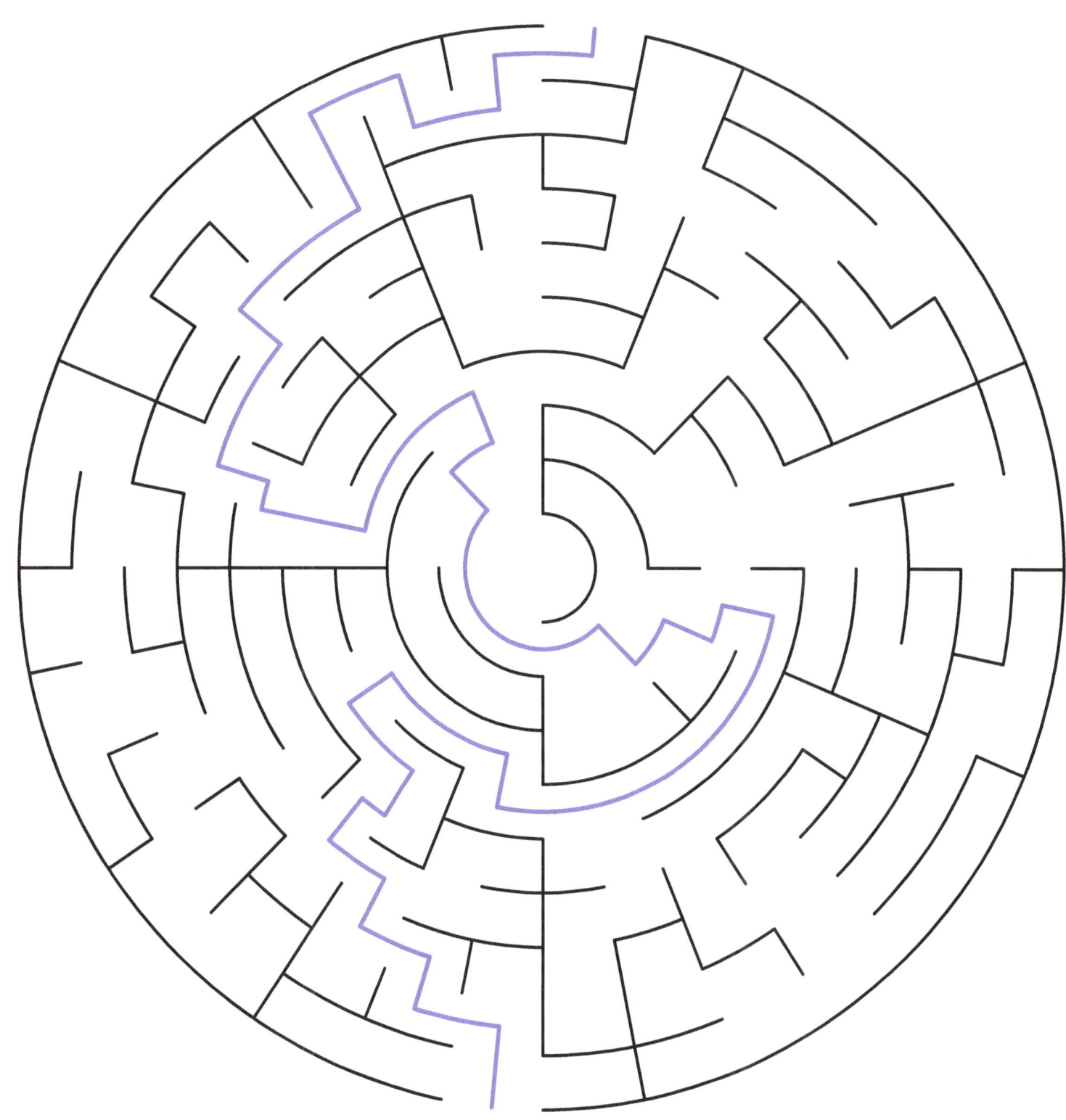

Maze Solution #4

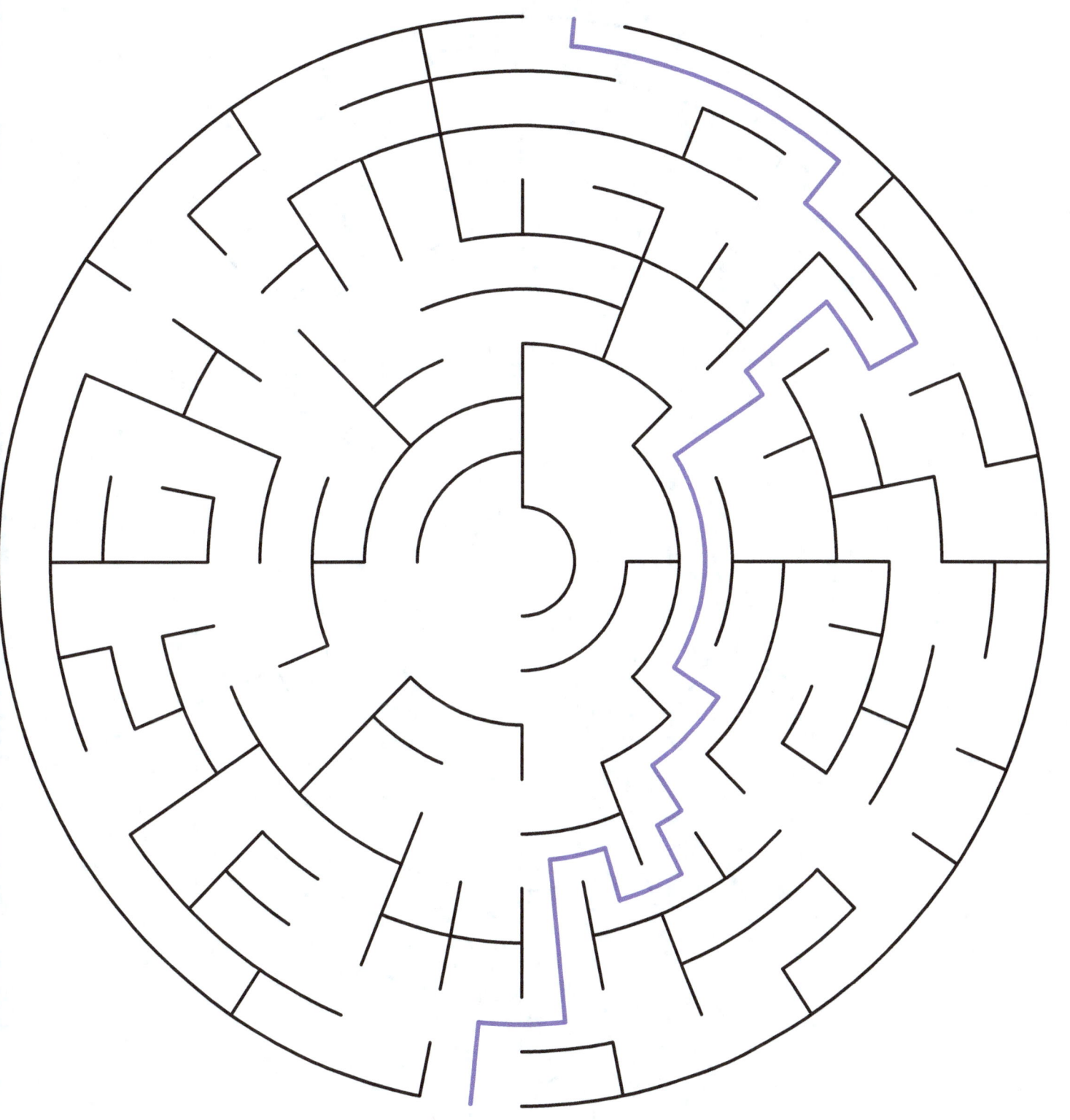

Maze Solution #5

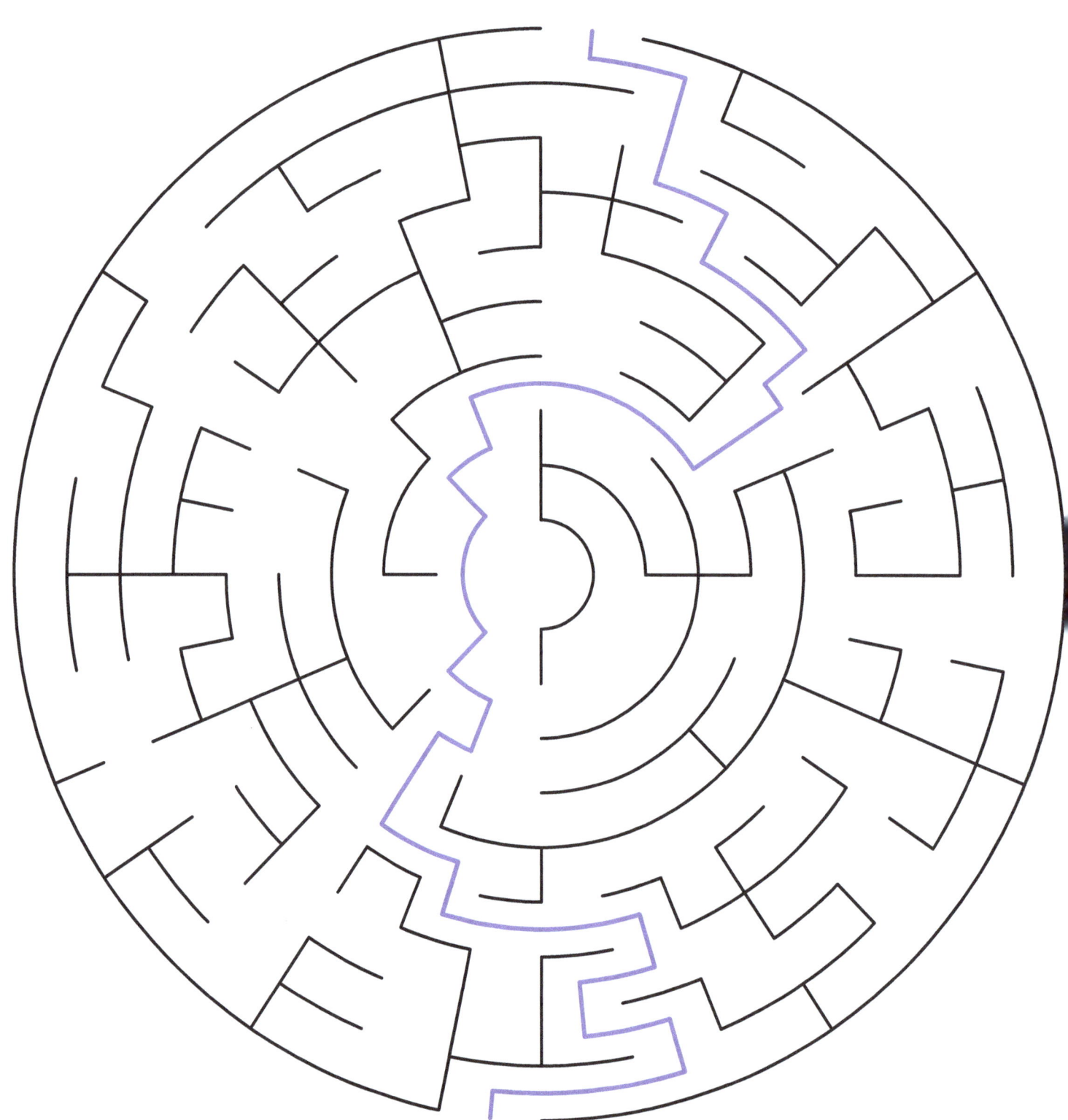

Maze Solution #6

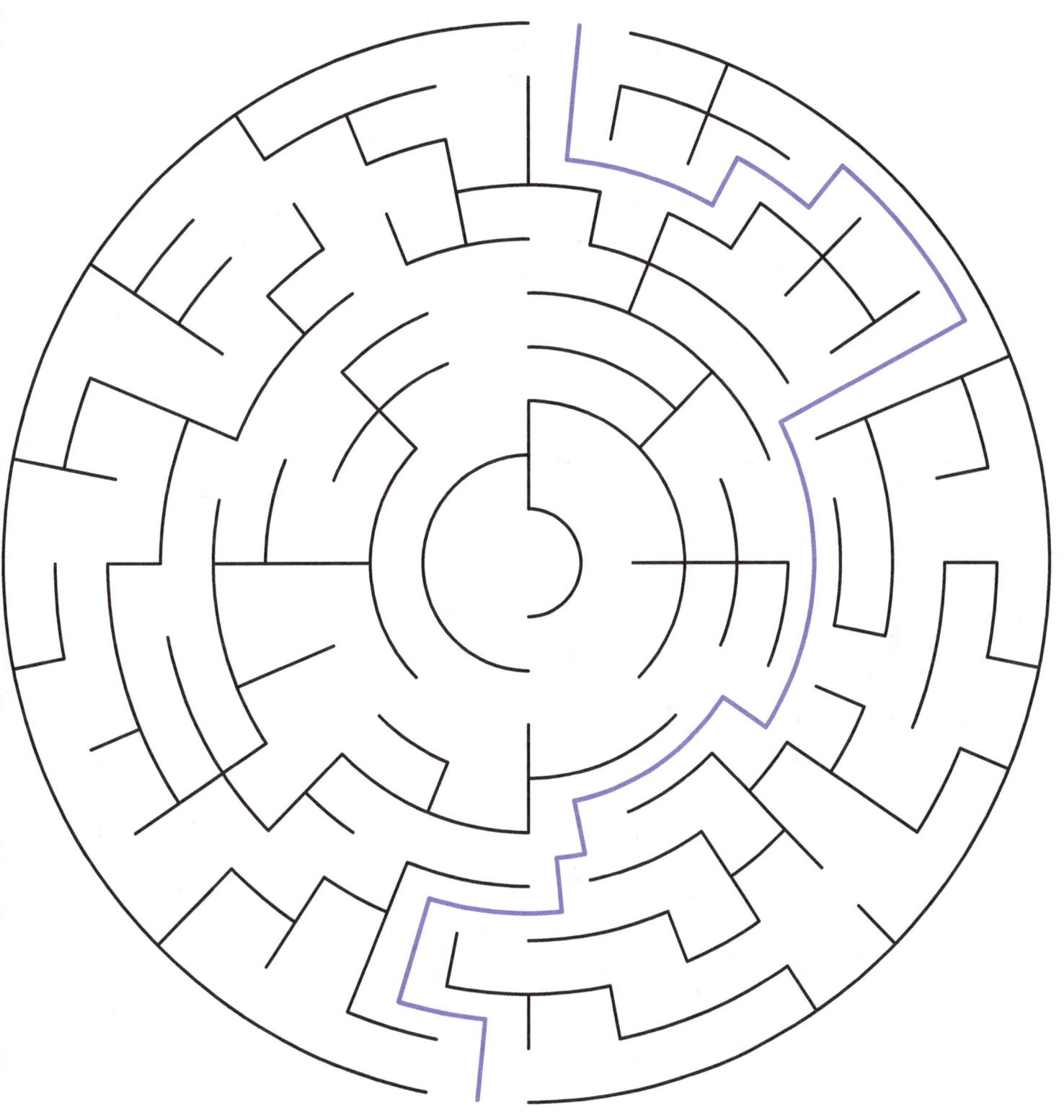

Maze Solution #7

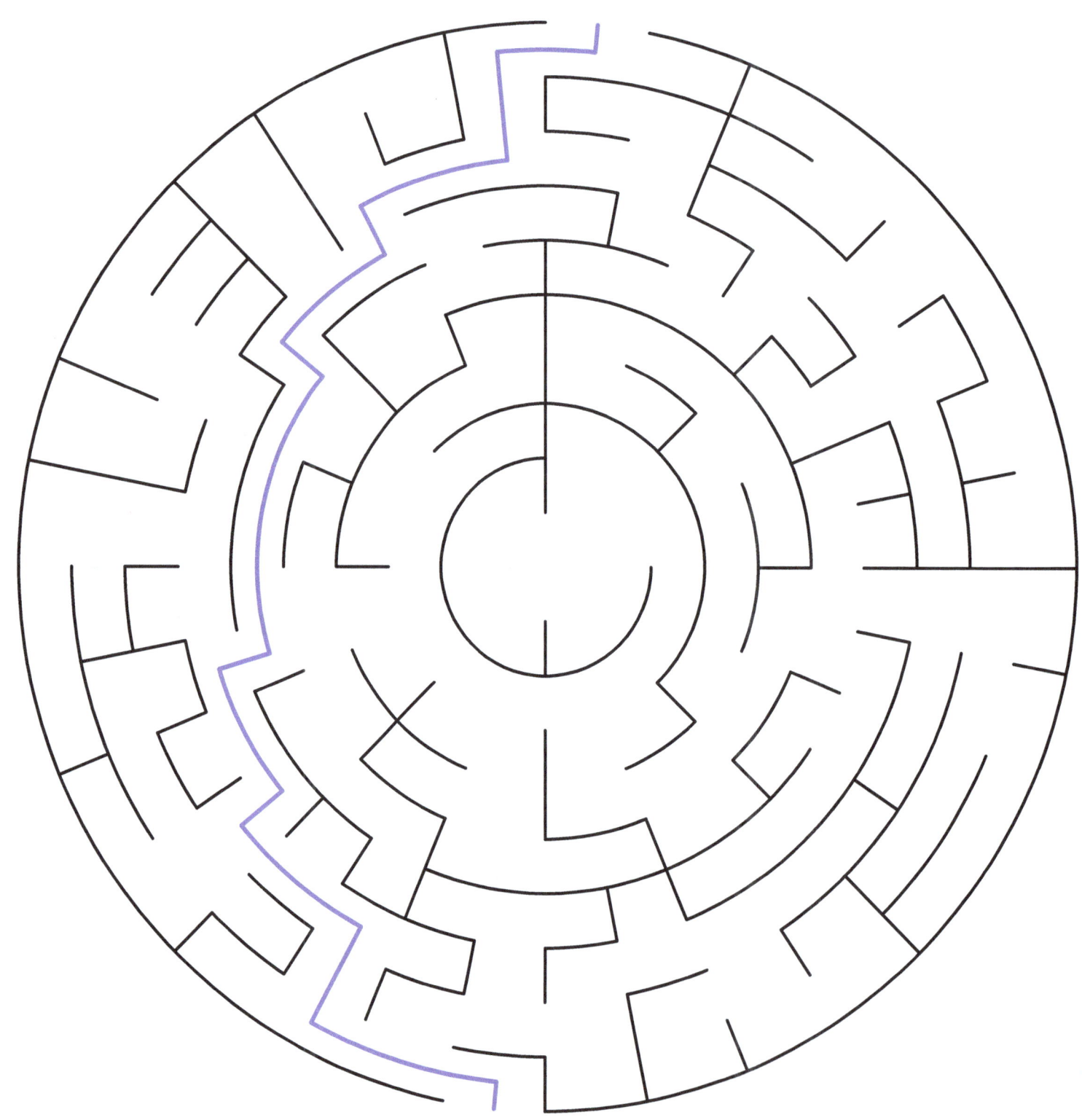

Maze Solution #8

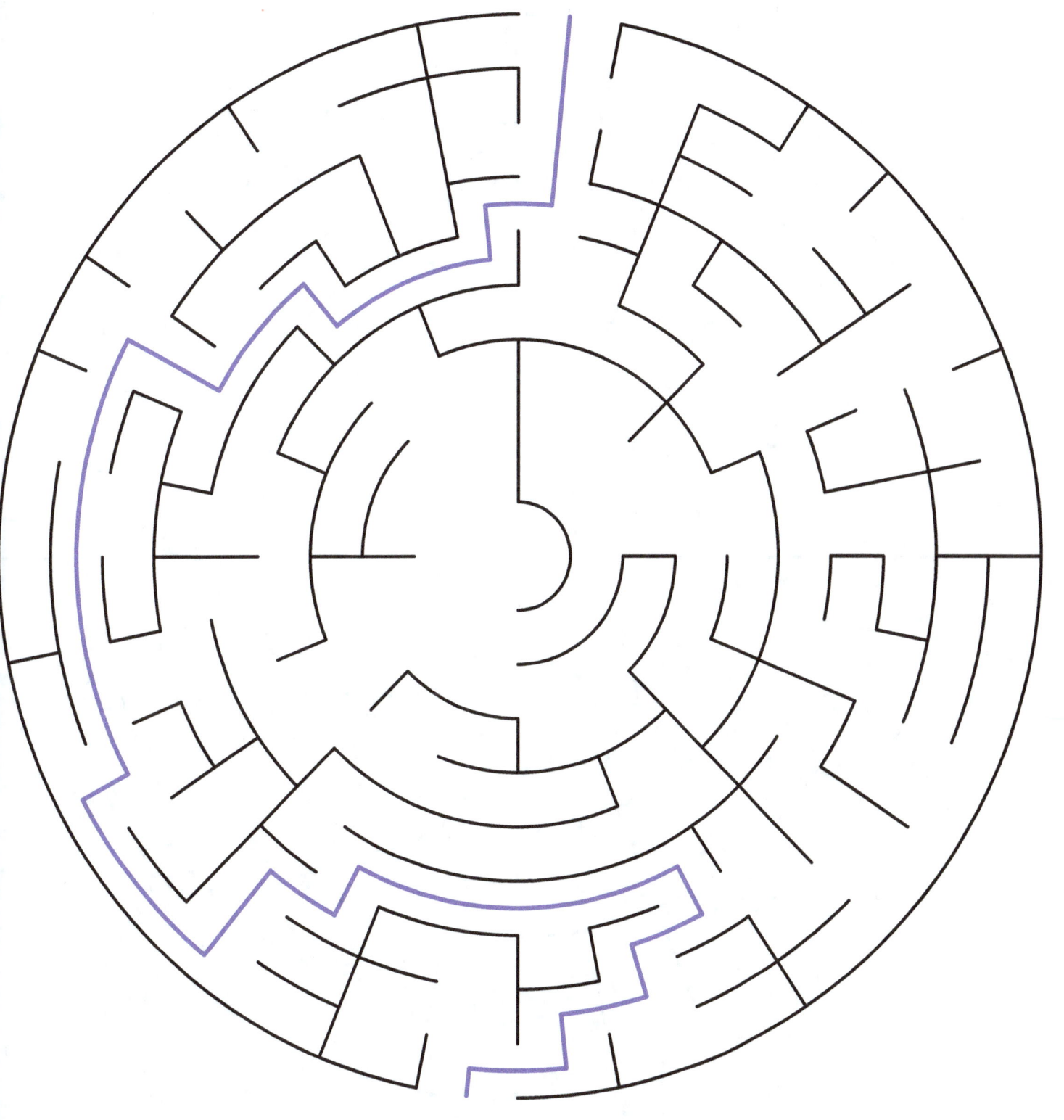

Maze Solution #9

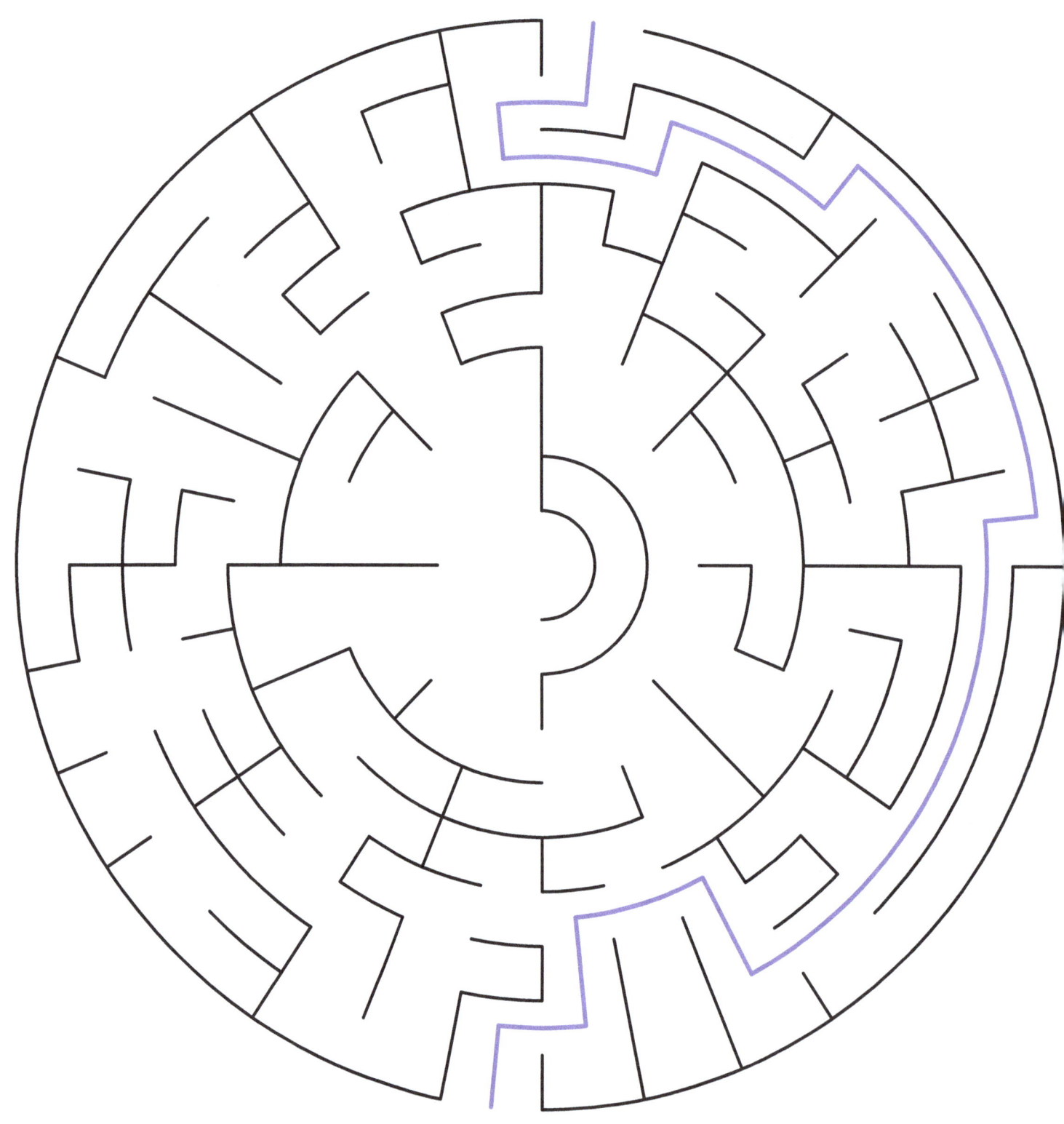

Maze Solution #10

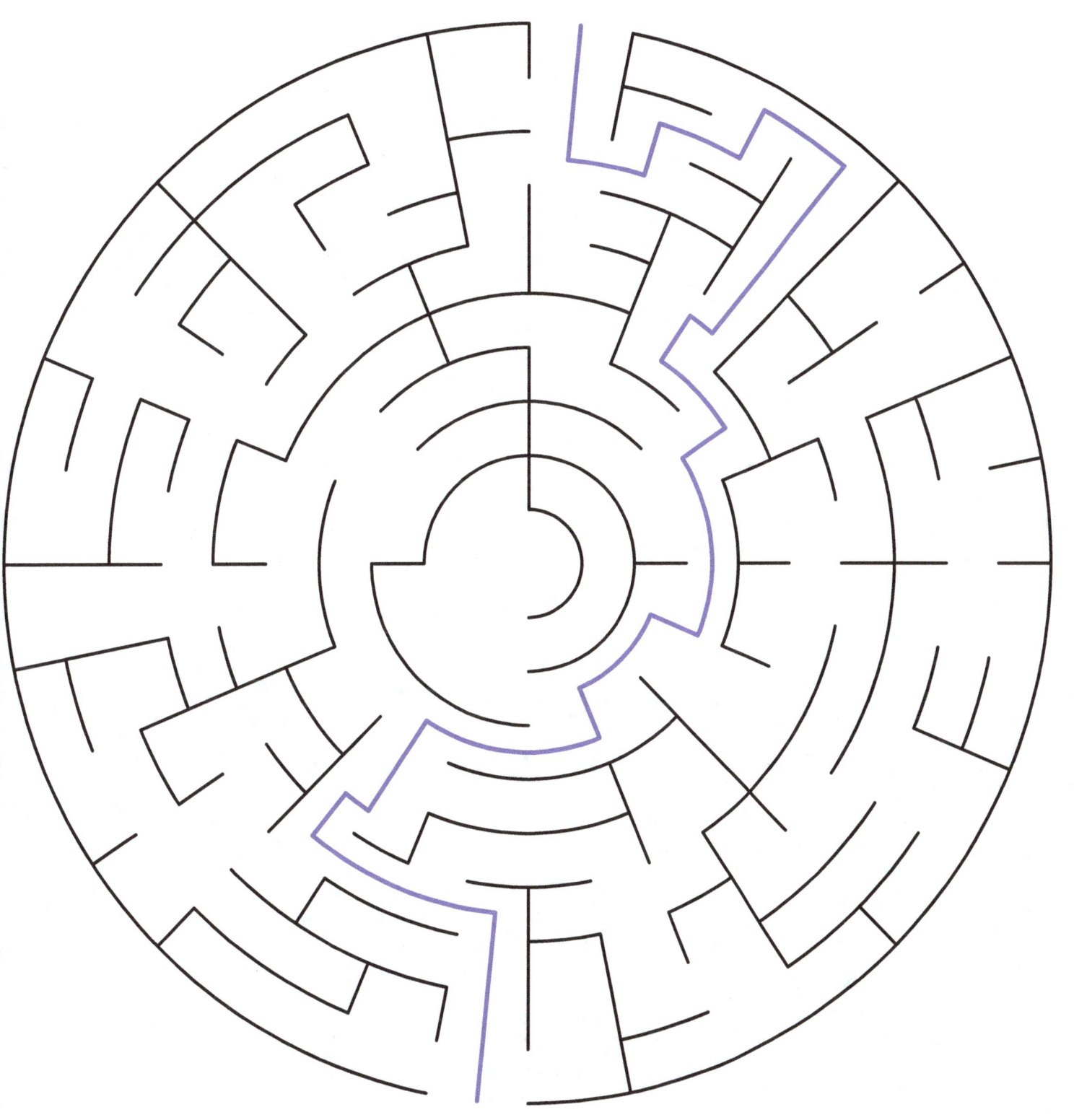

Maze Solution #11

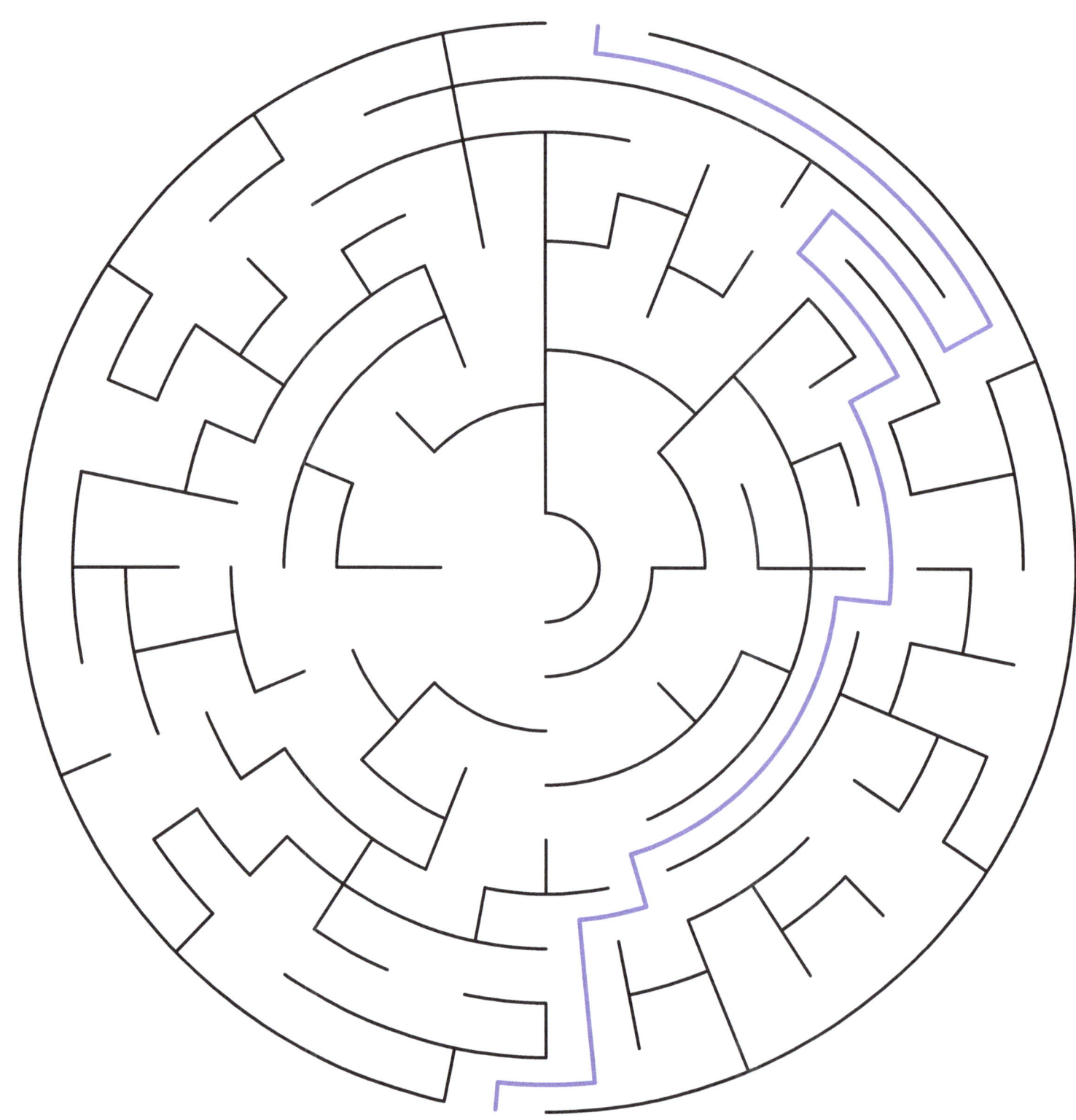

Maze Solution #12

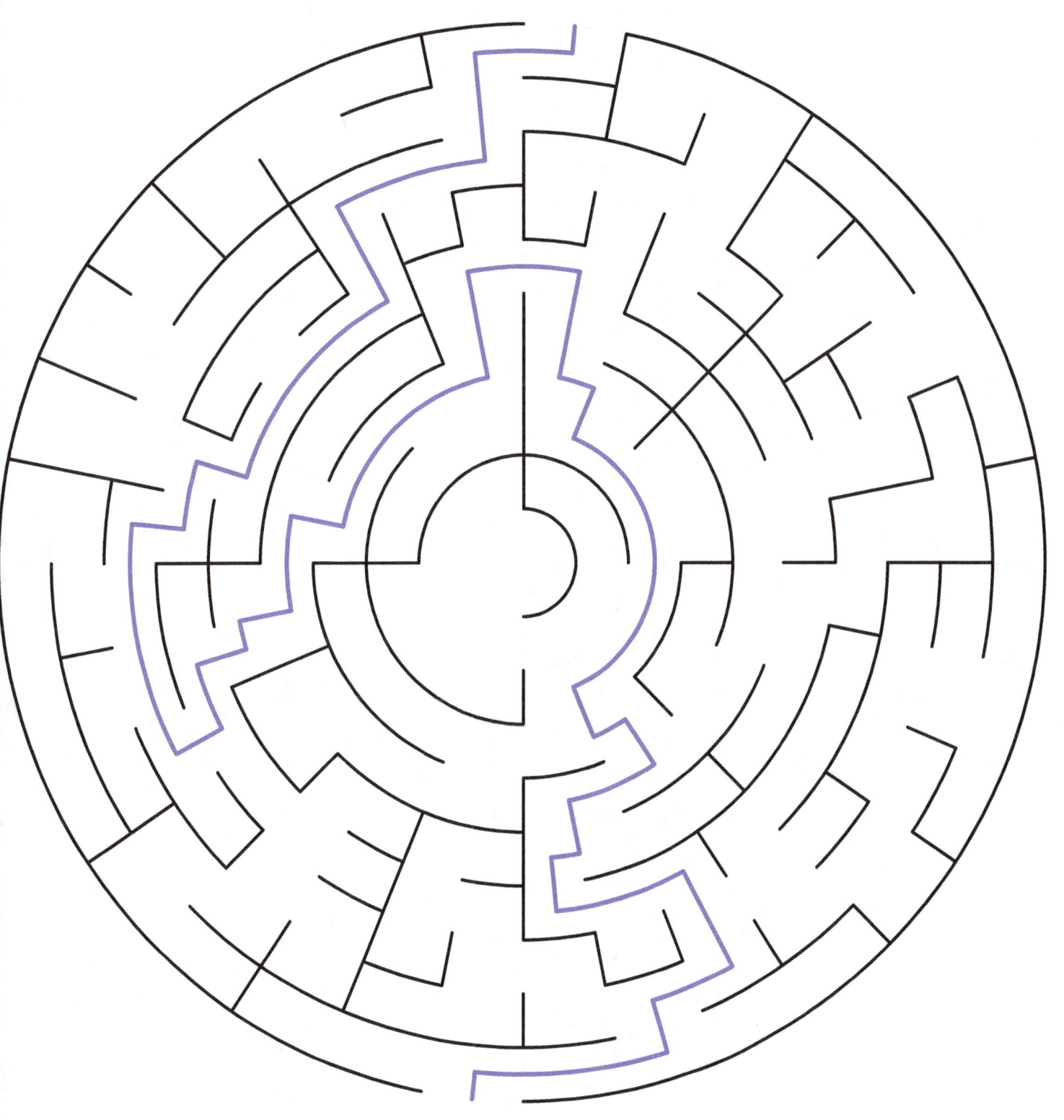

Maze Solution #13

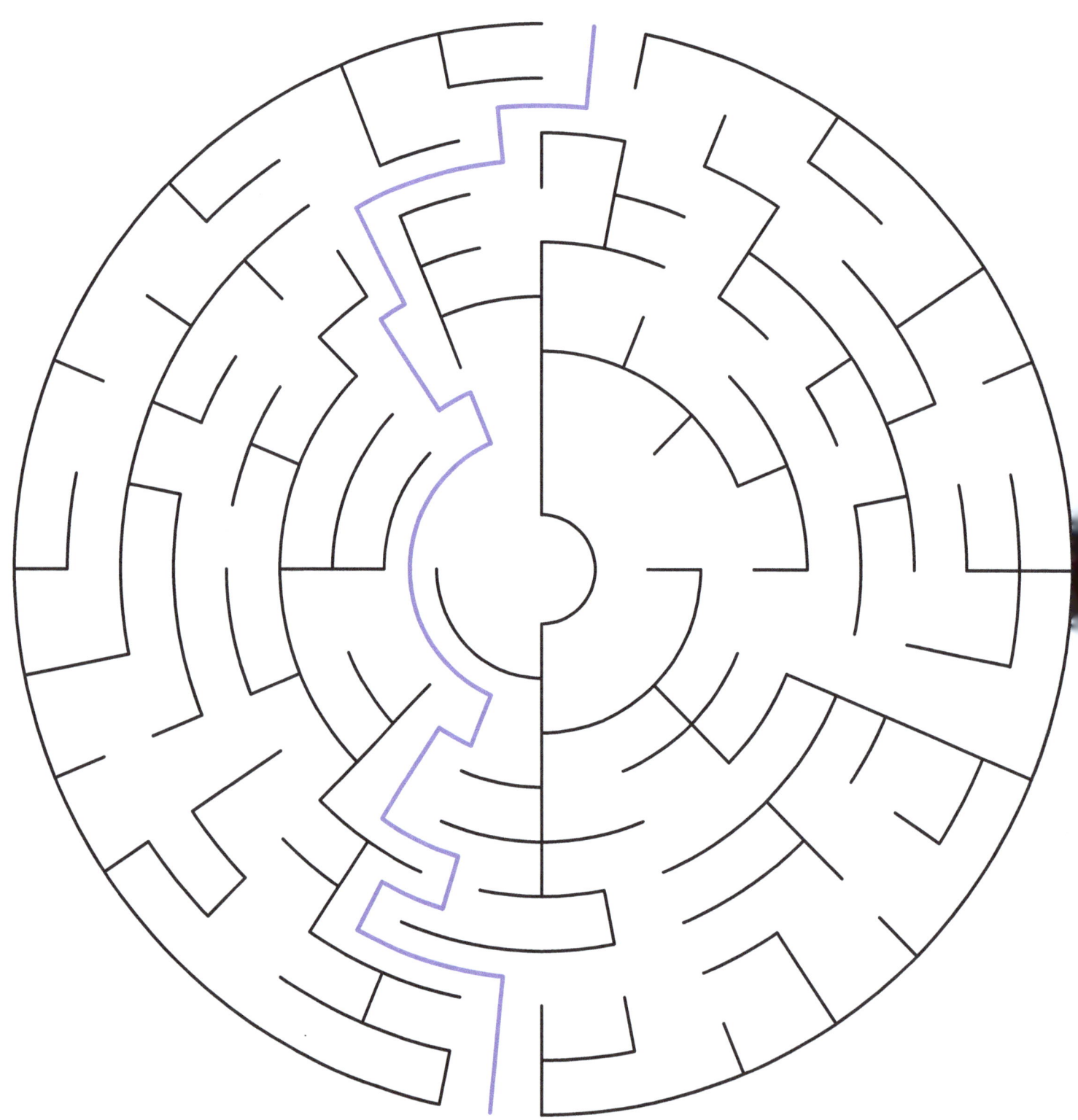

Maze Solution #14

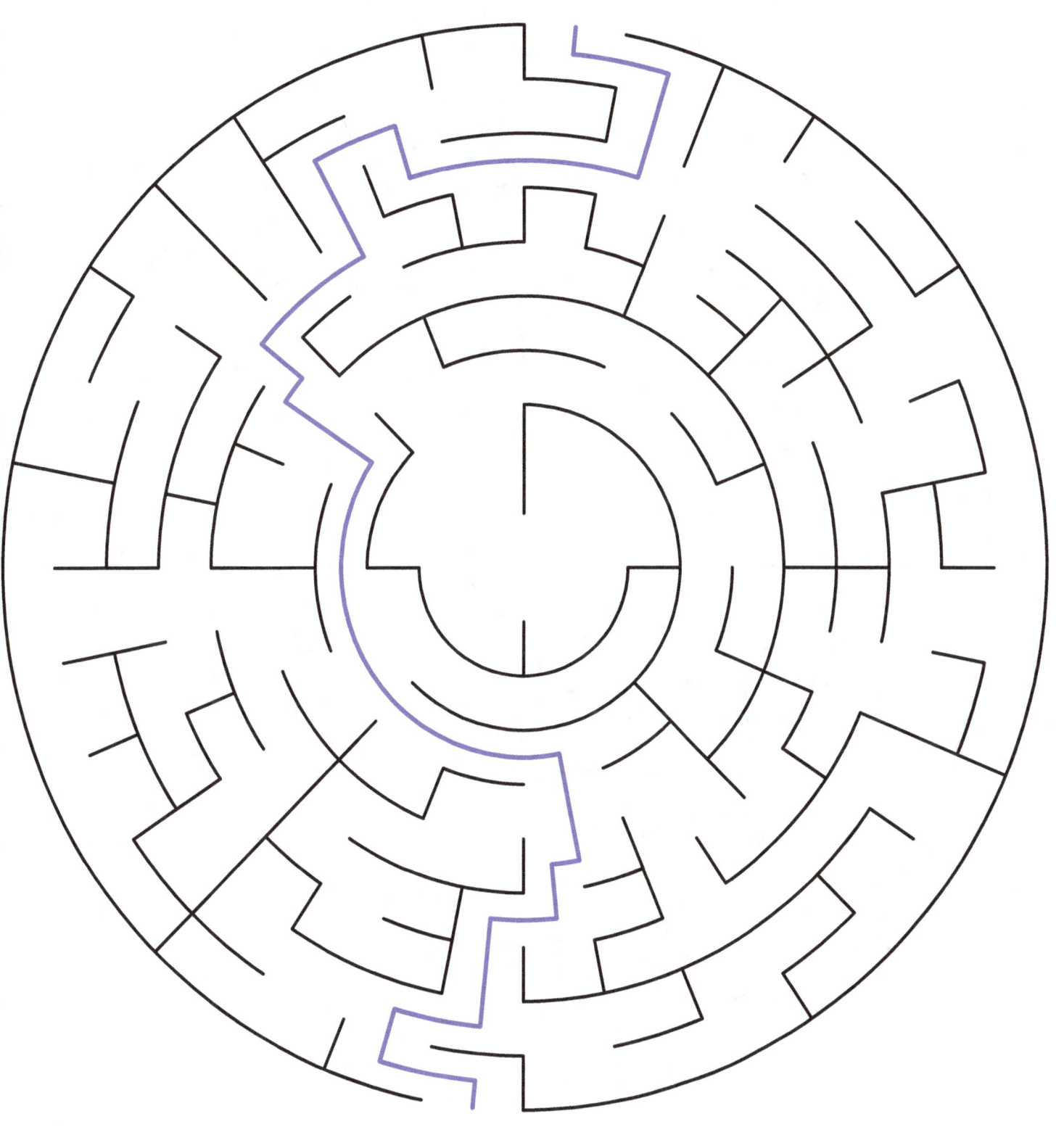

Maze Solution #15

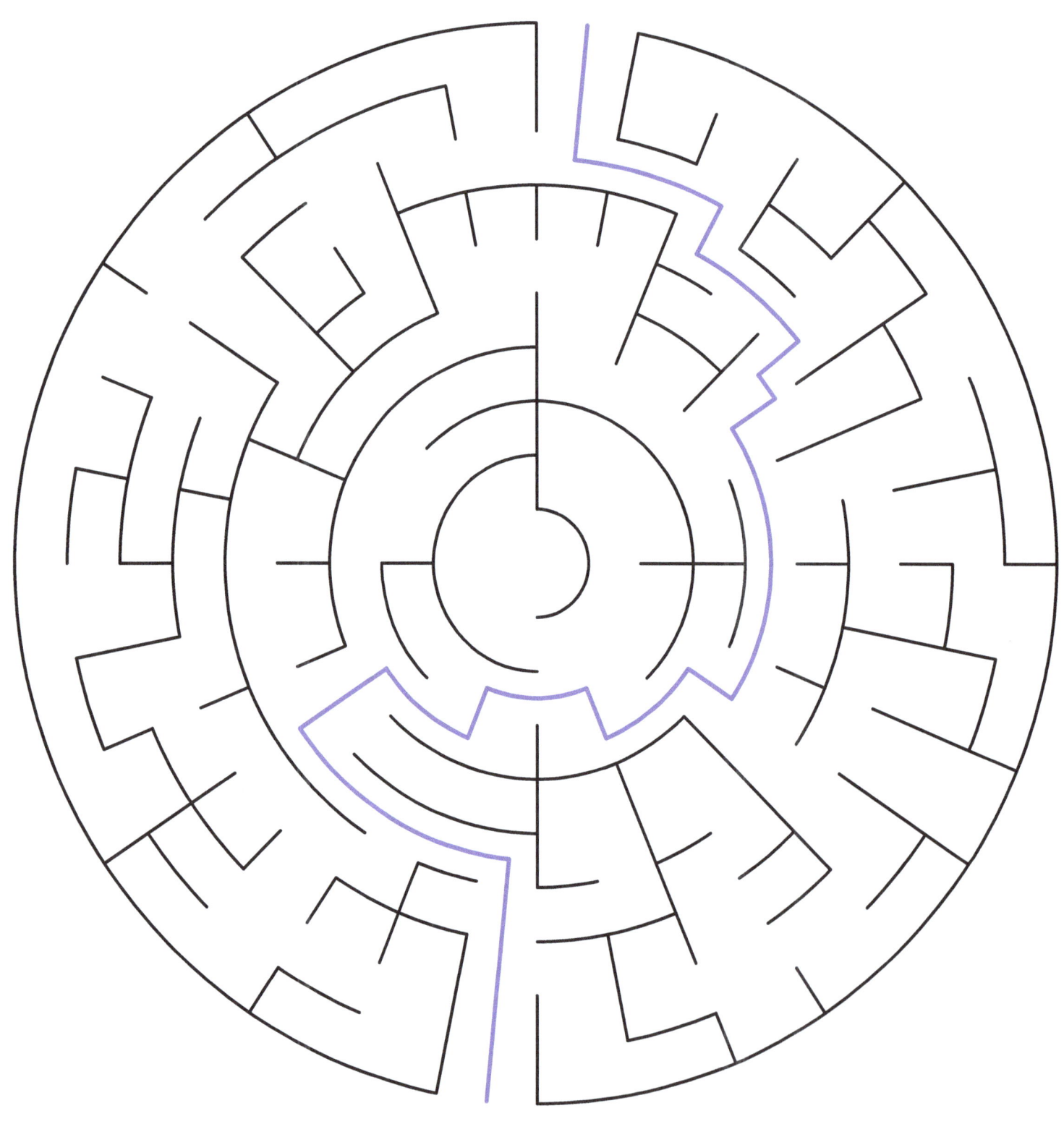

Maze Solution #16

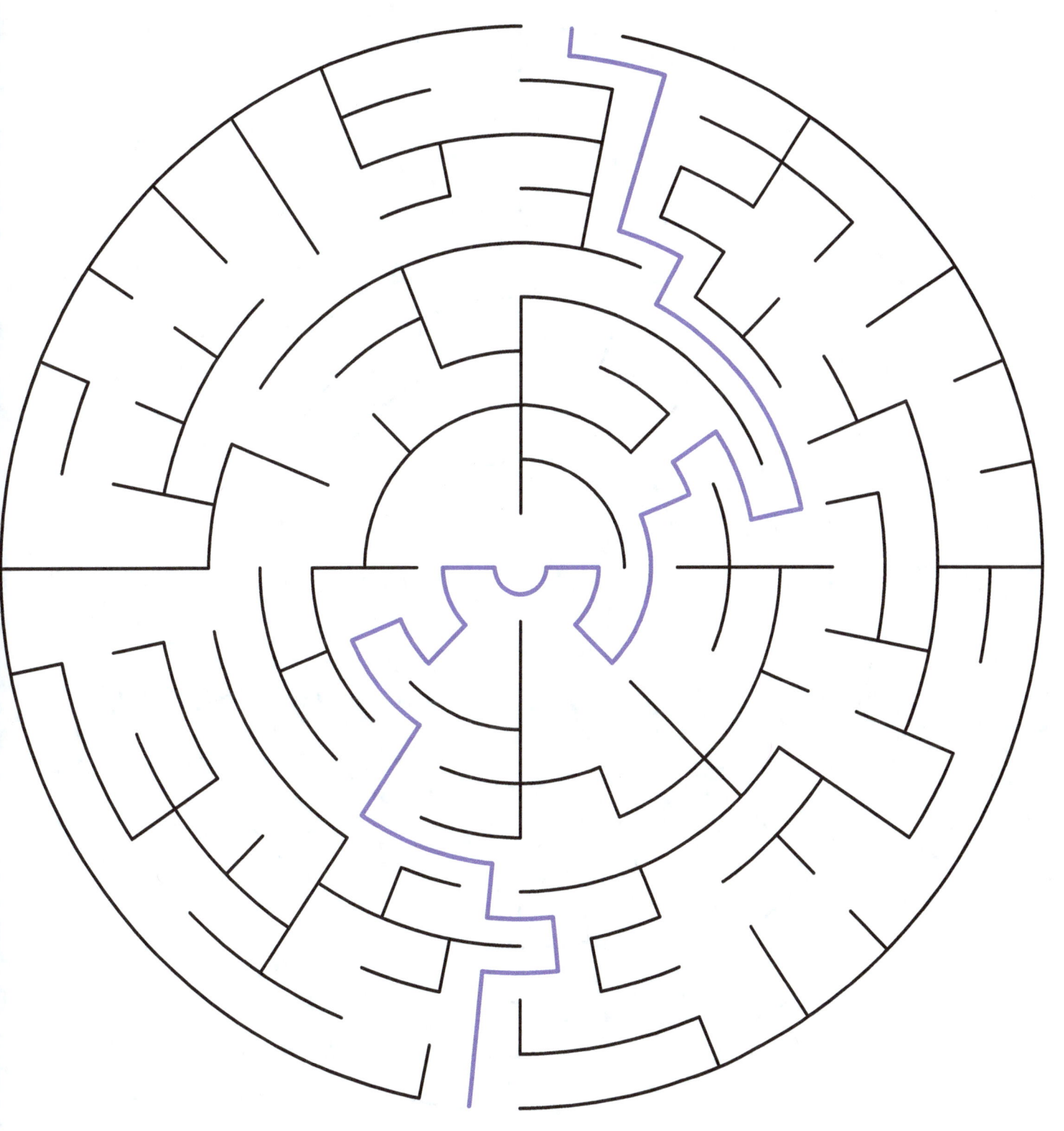

Maze Solution #17

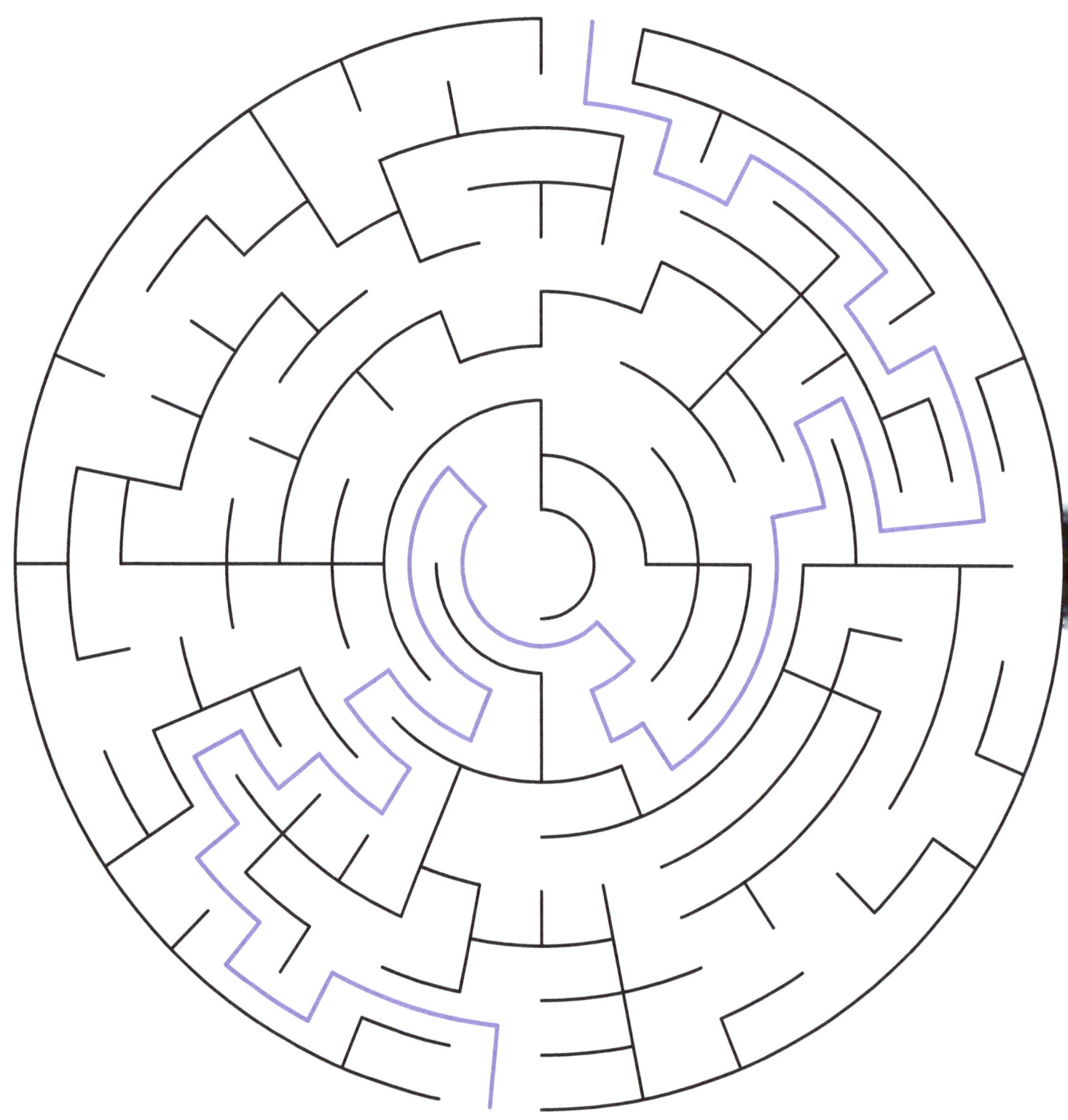

Maze Solution #18

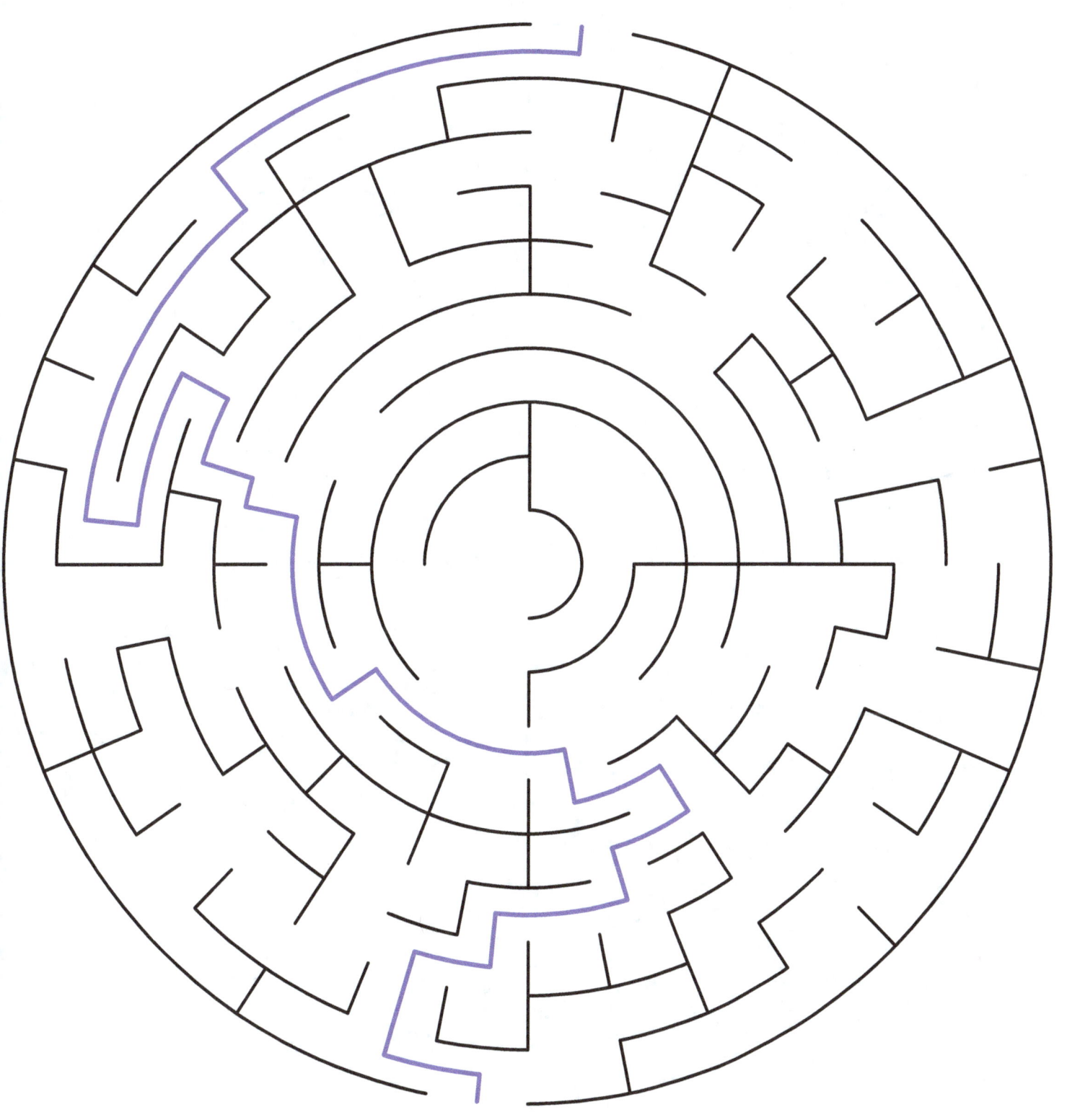

Maze Solution #19

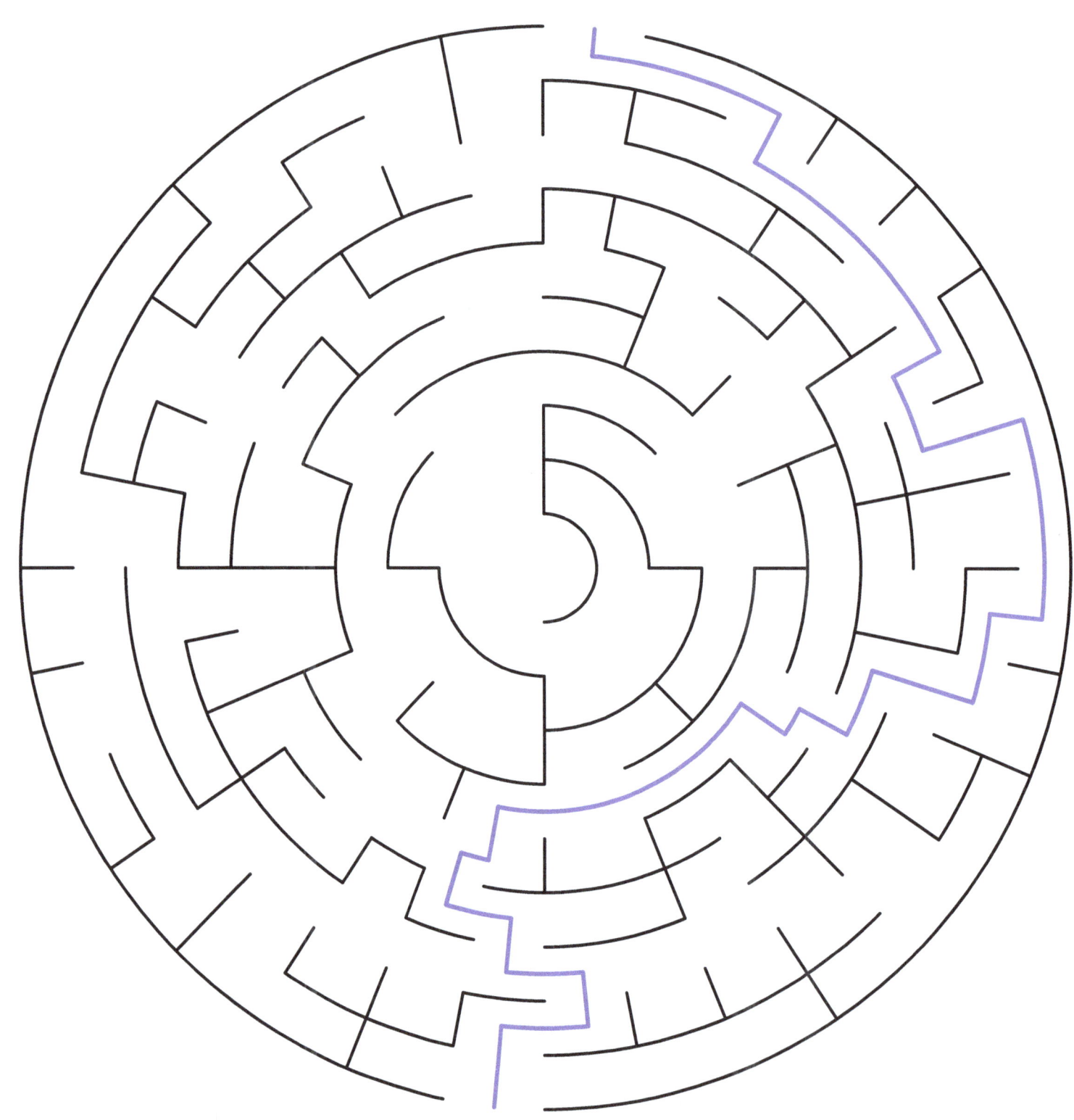

Maze Solution #20

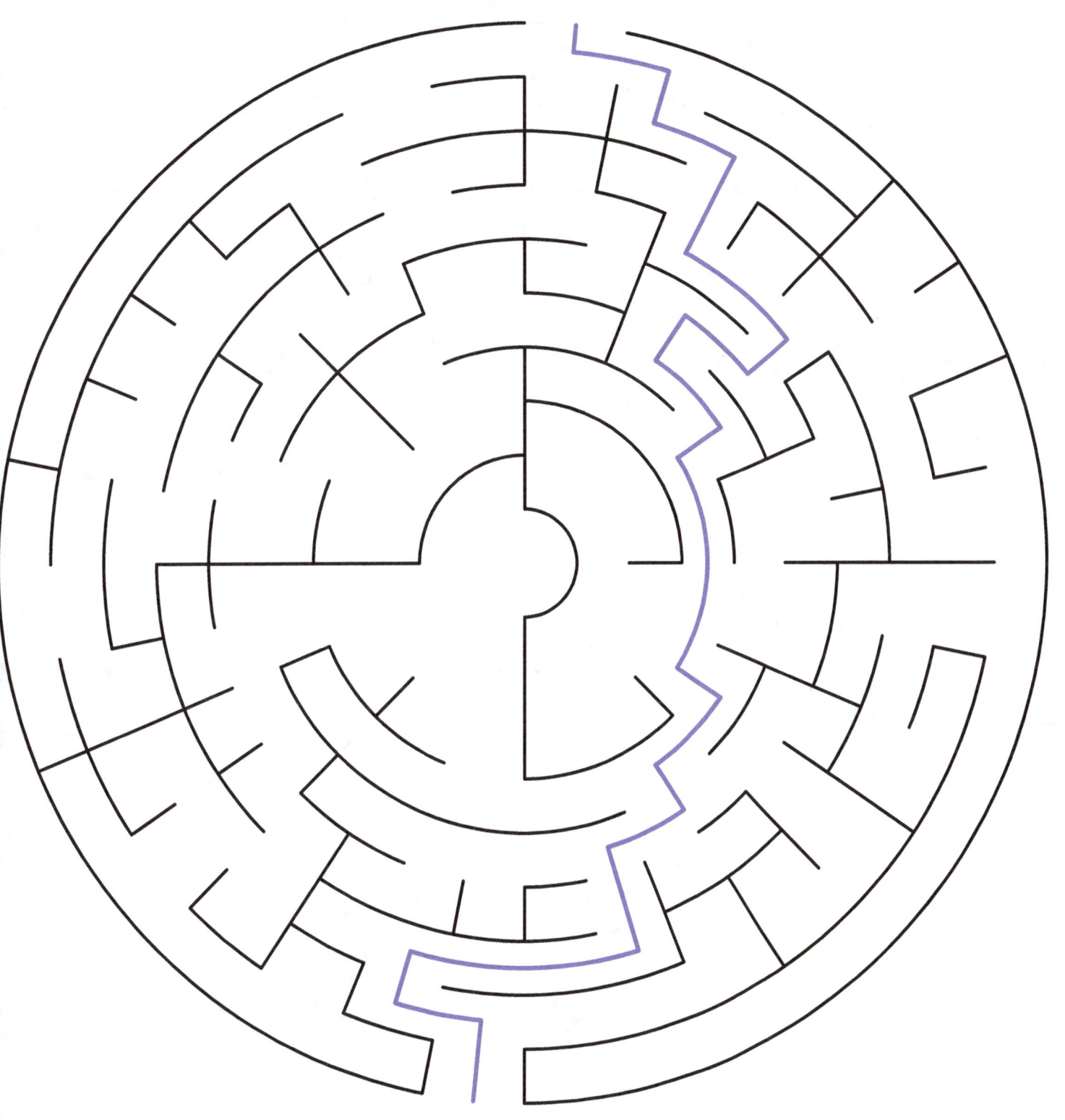

Maze Solution #21

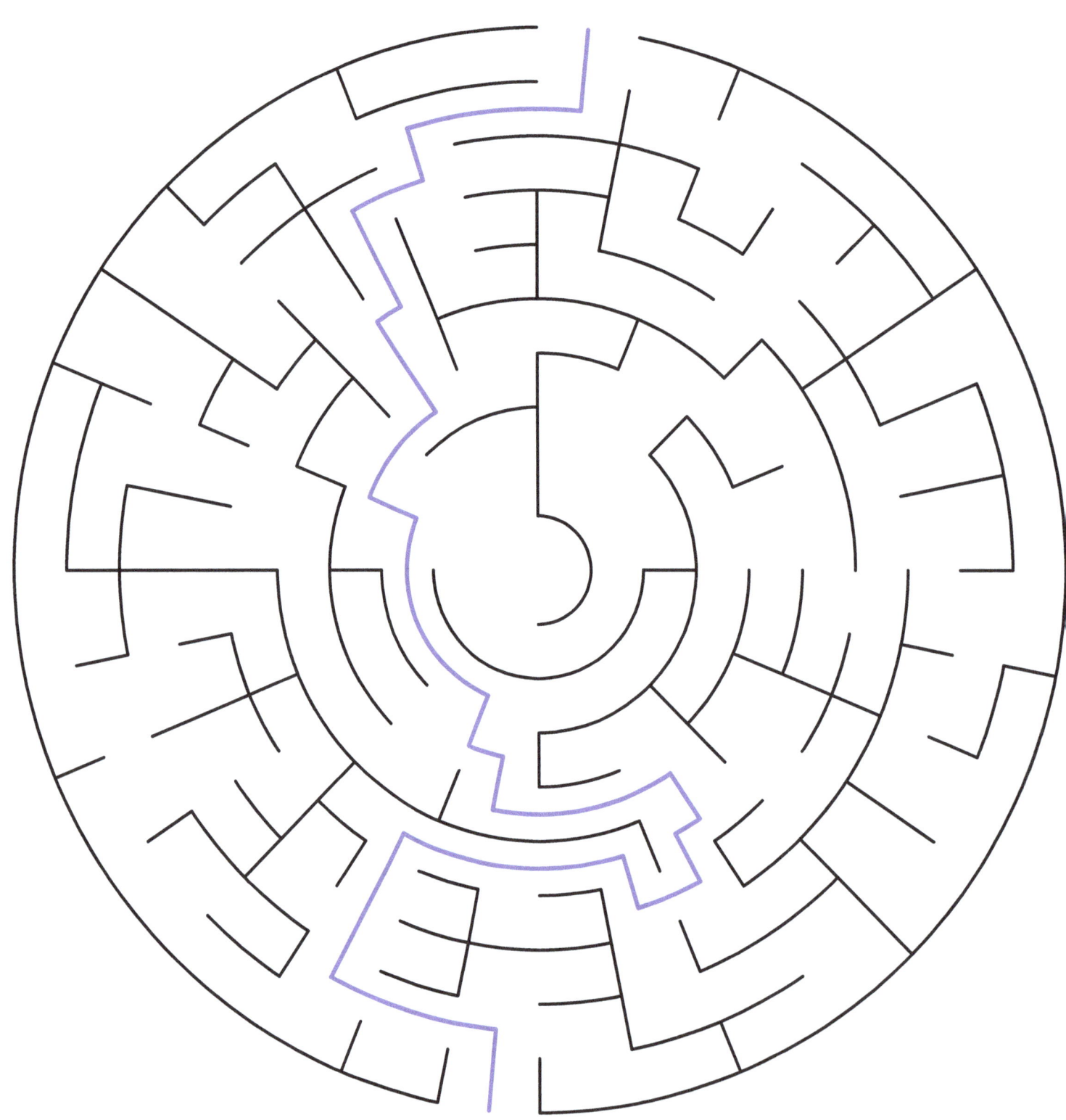

Maze Solution #22

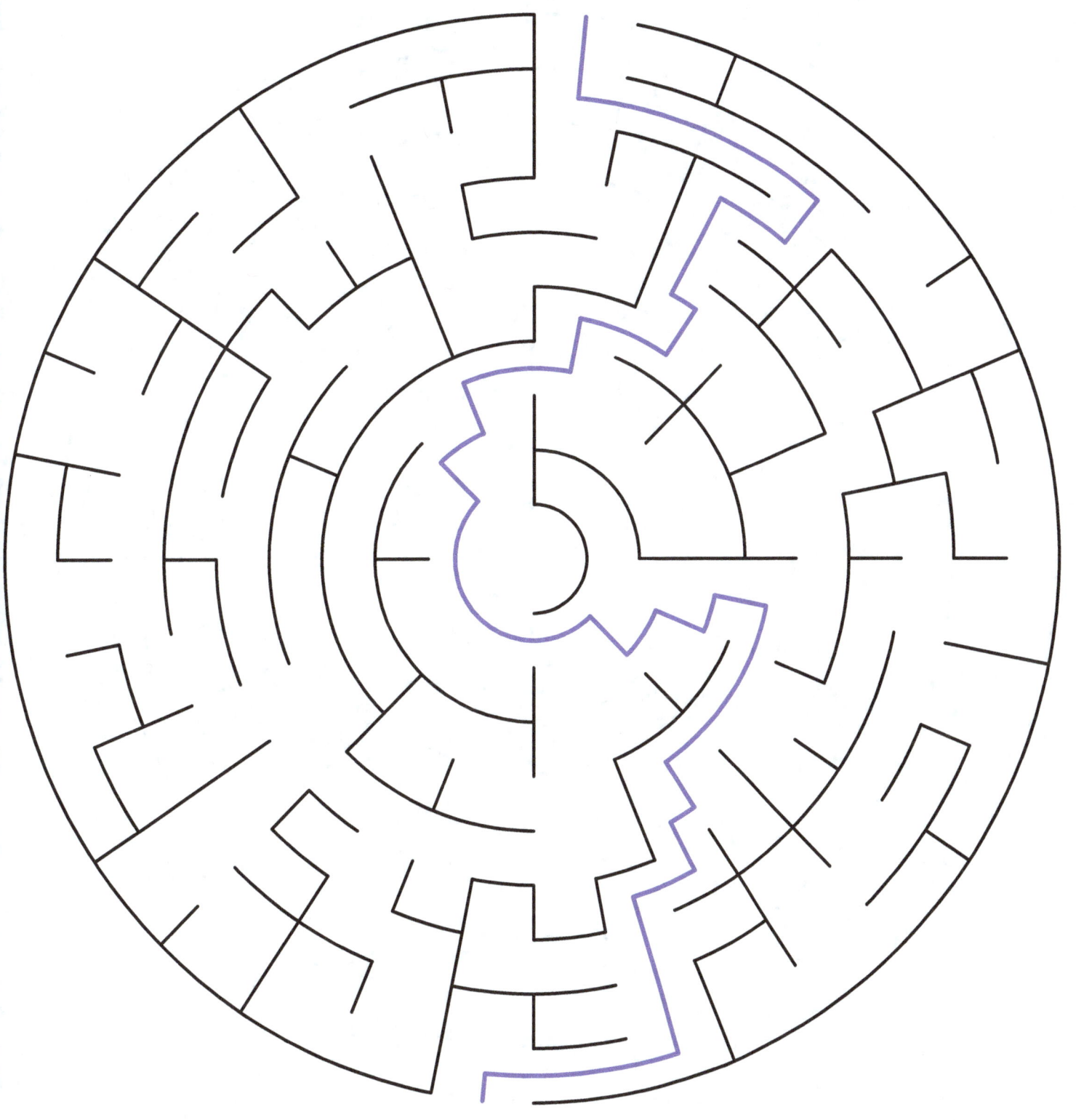

Maze Solution #23

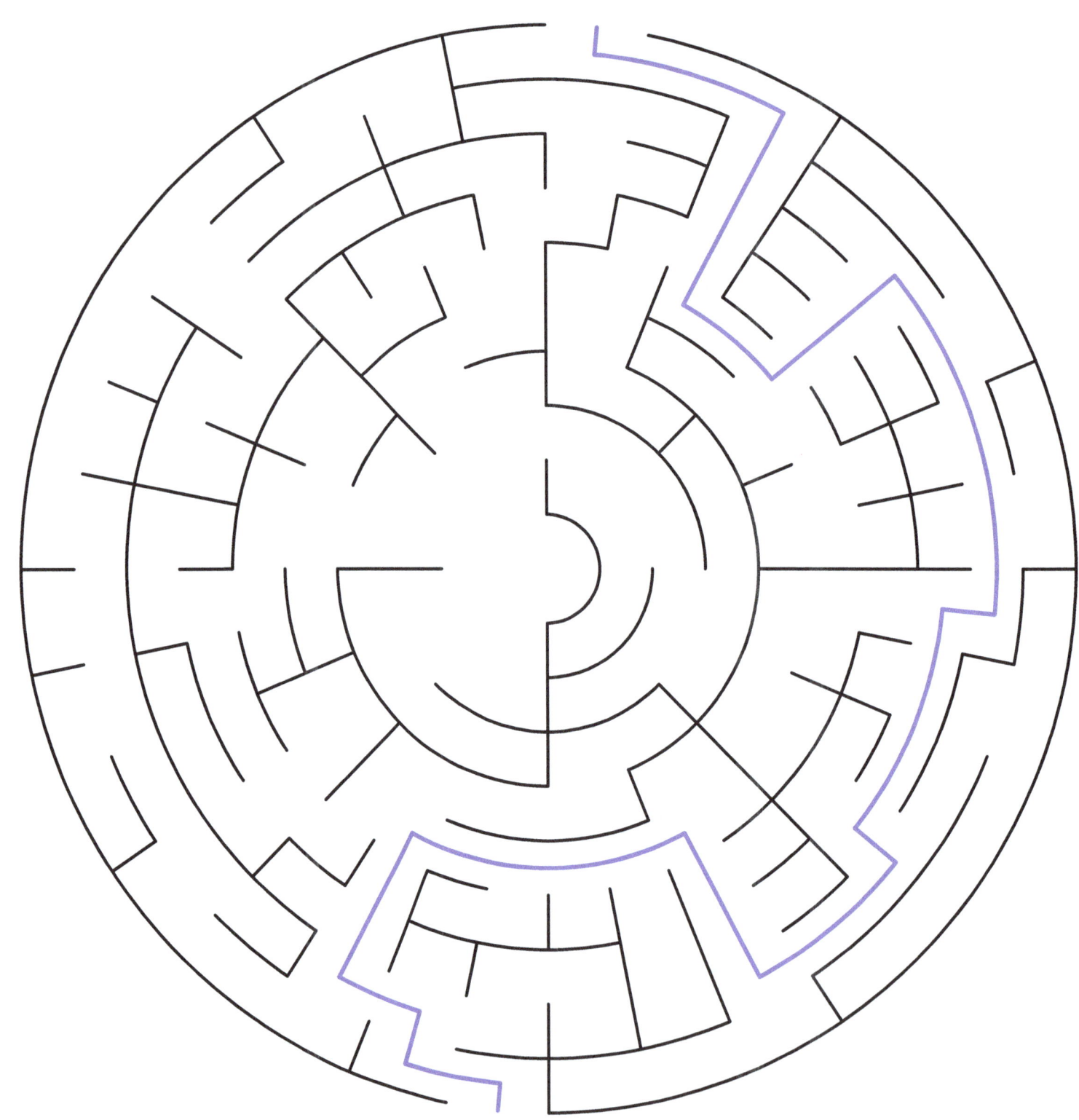

Maze Solution #24

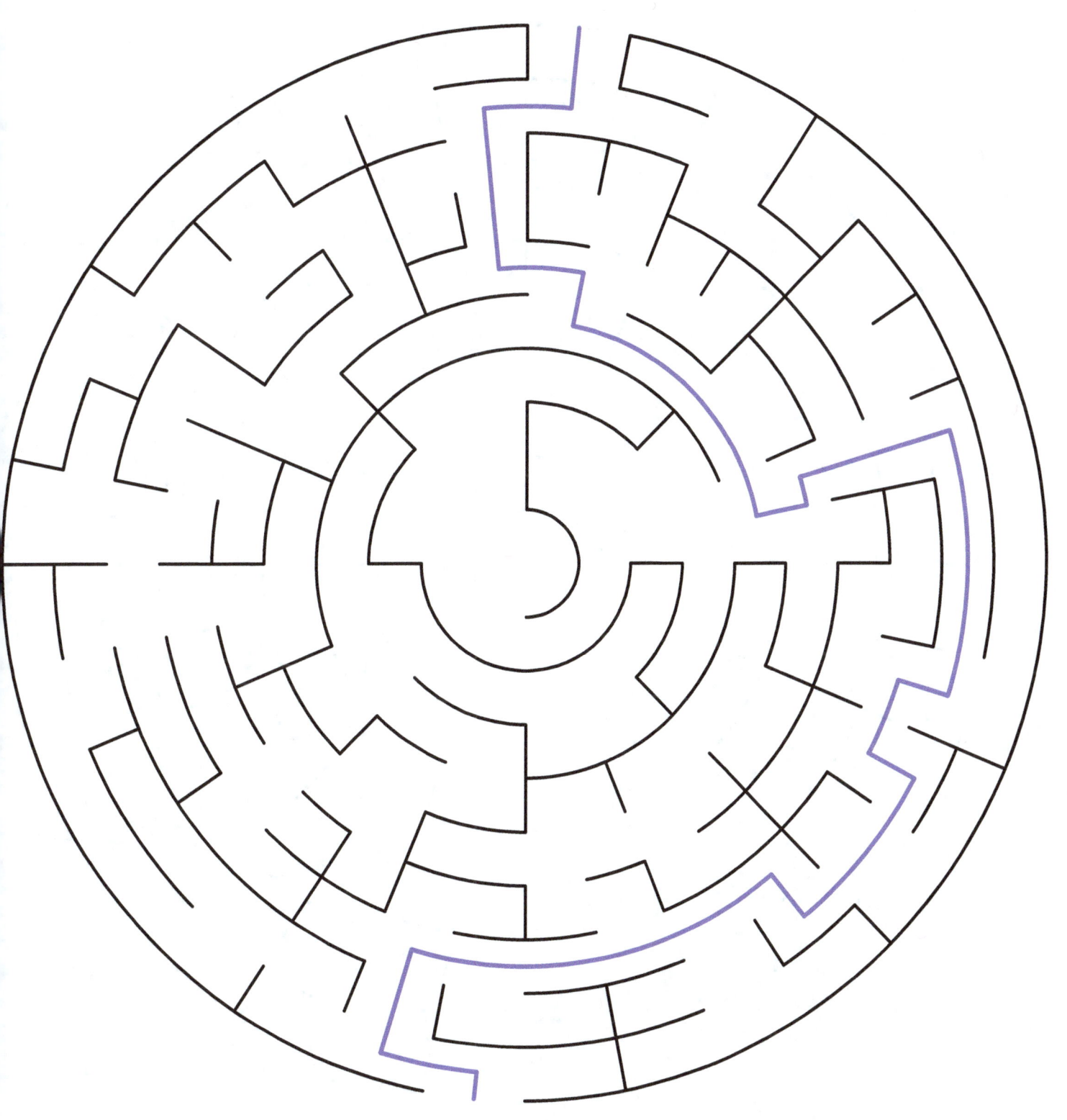

Maze Solution #25

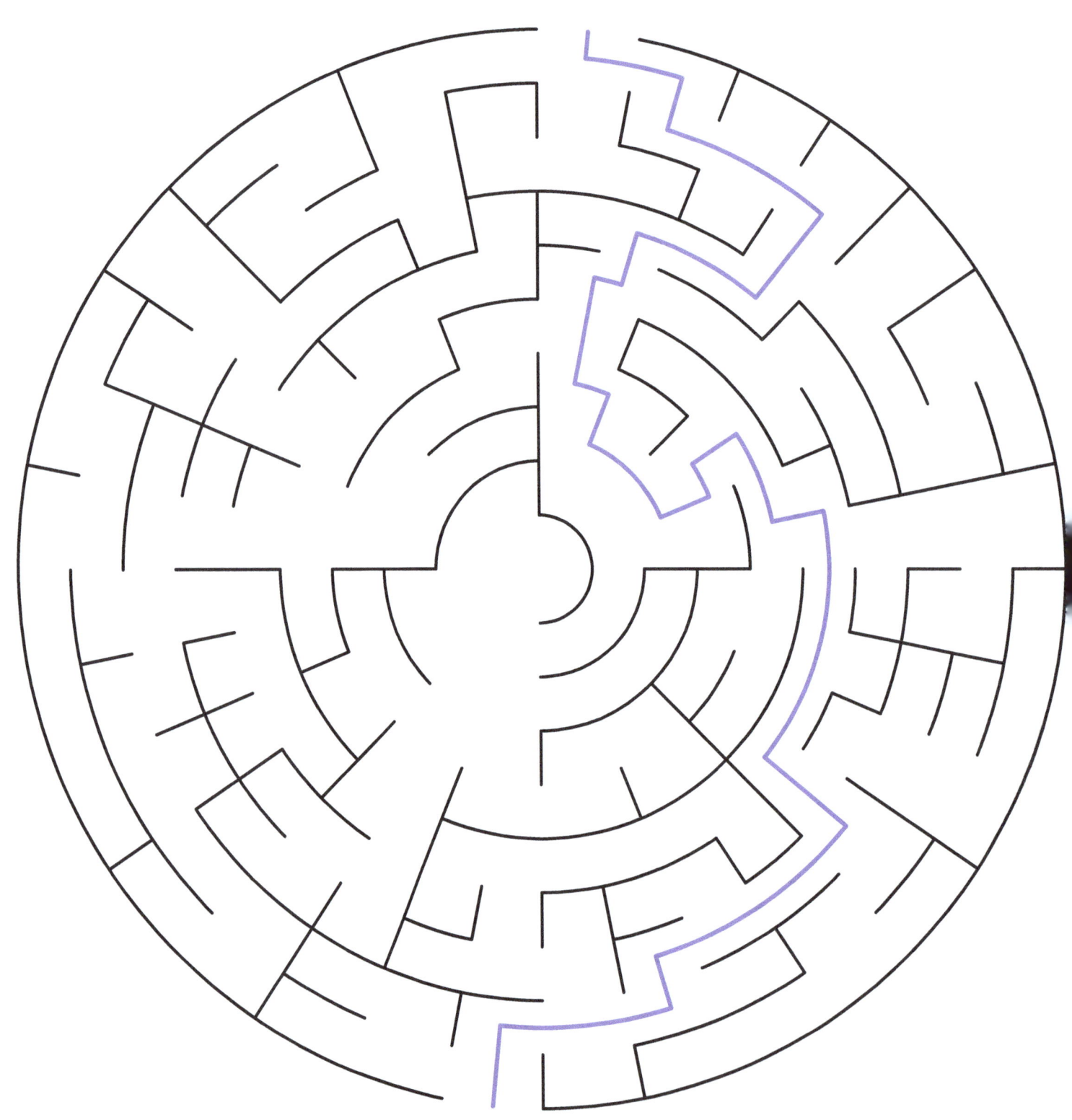

Maze Solution #26

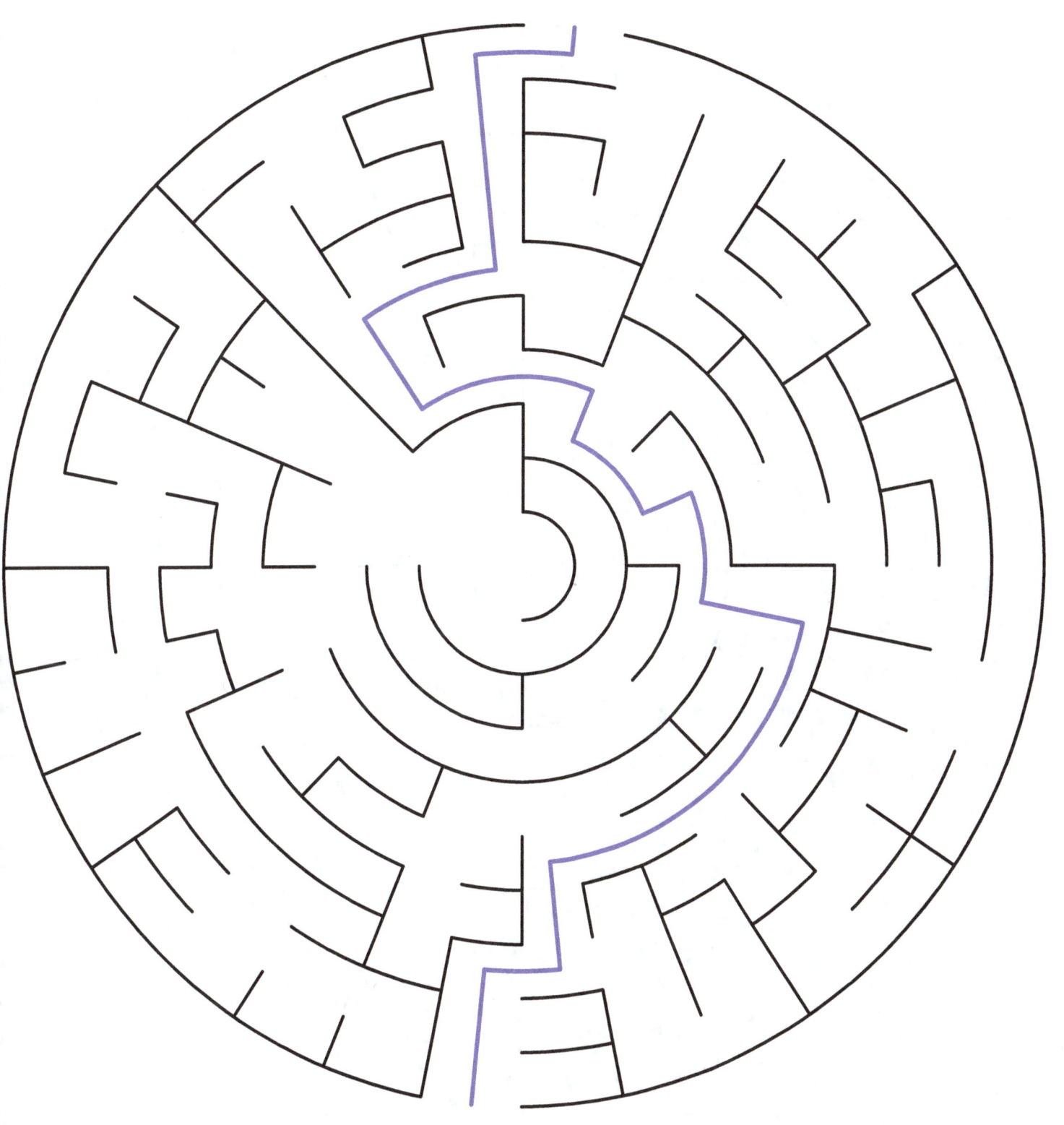

Maze Solution #27

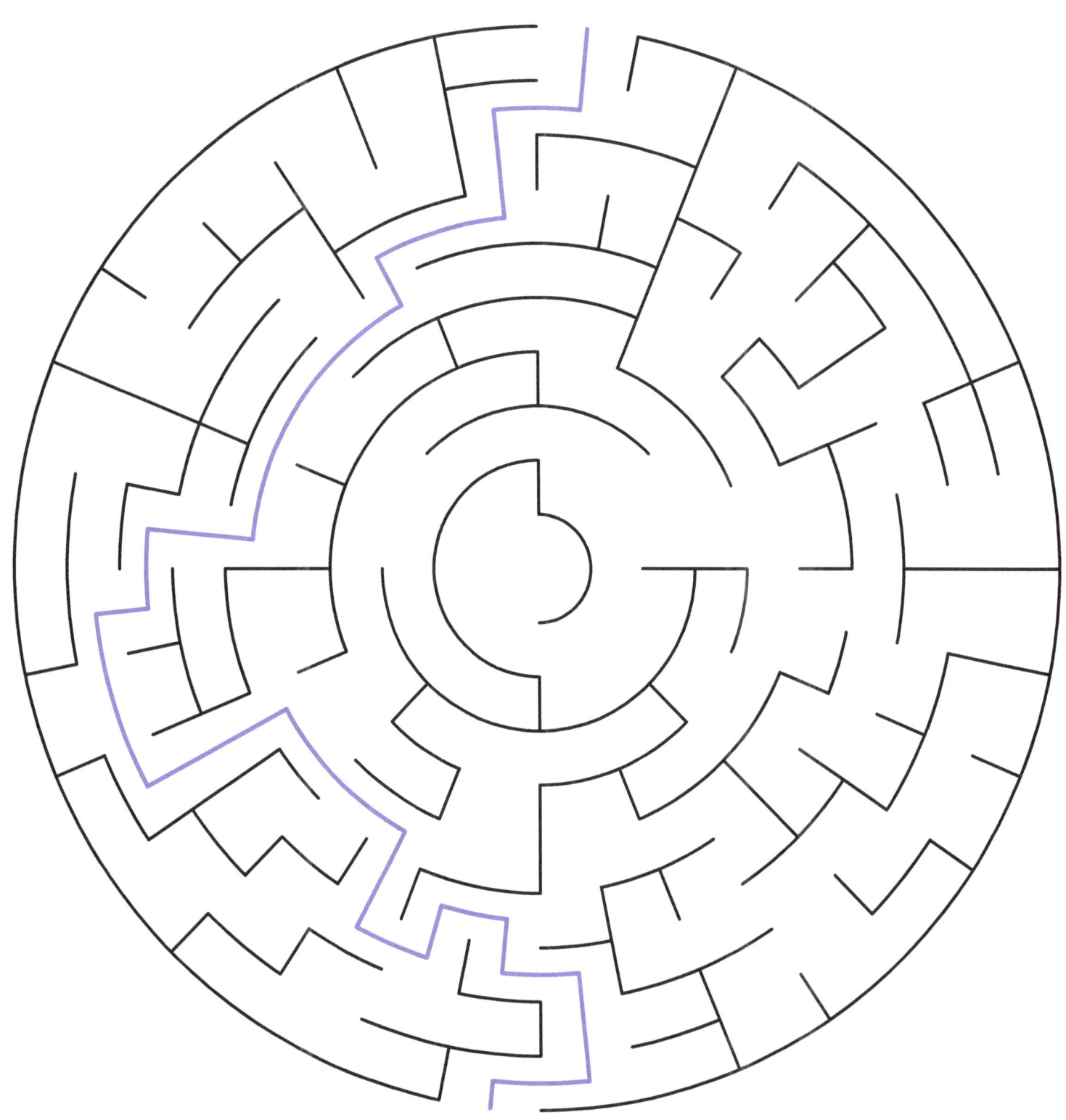

Maze Solution #28

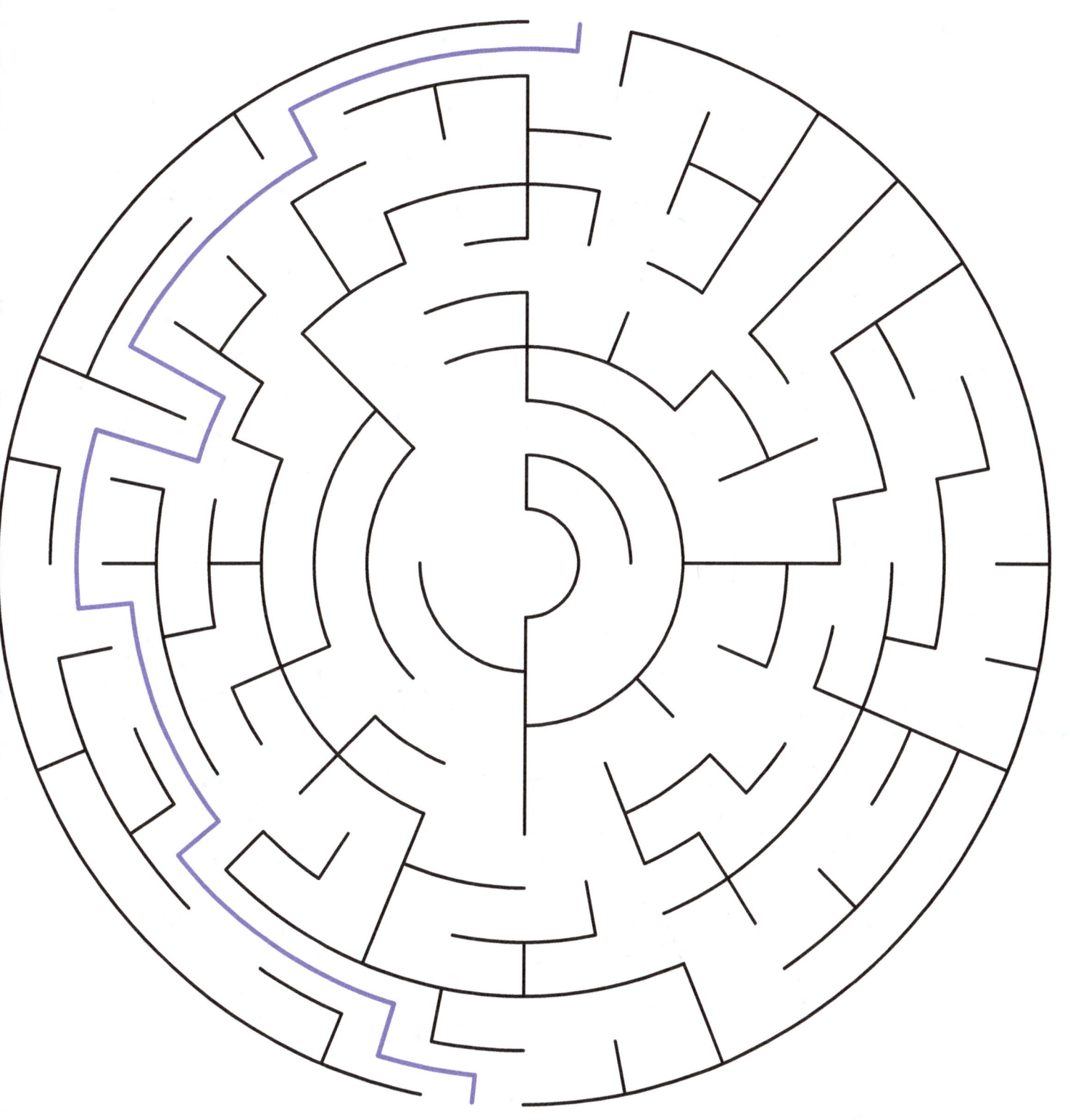

Maze Solution #29

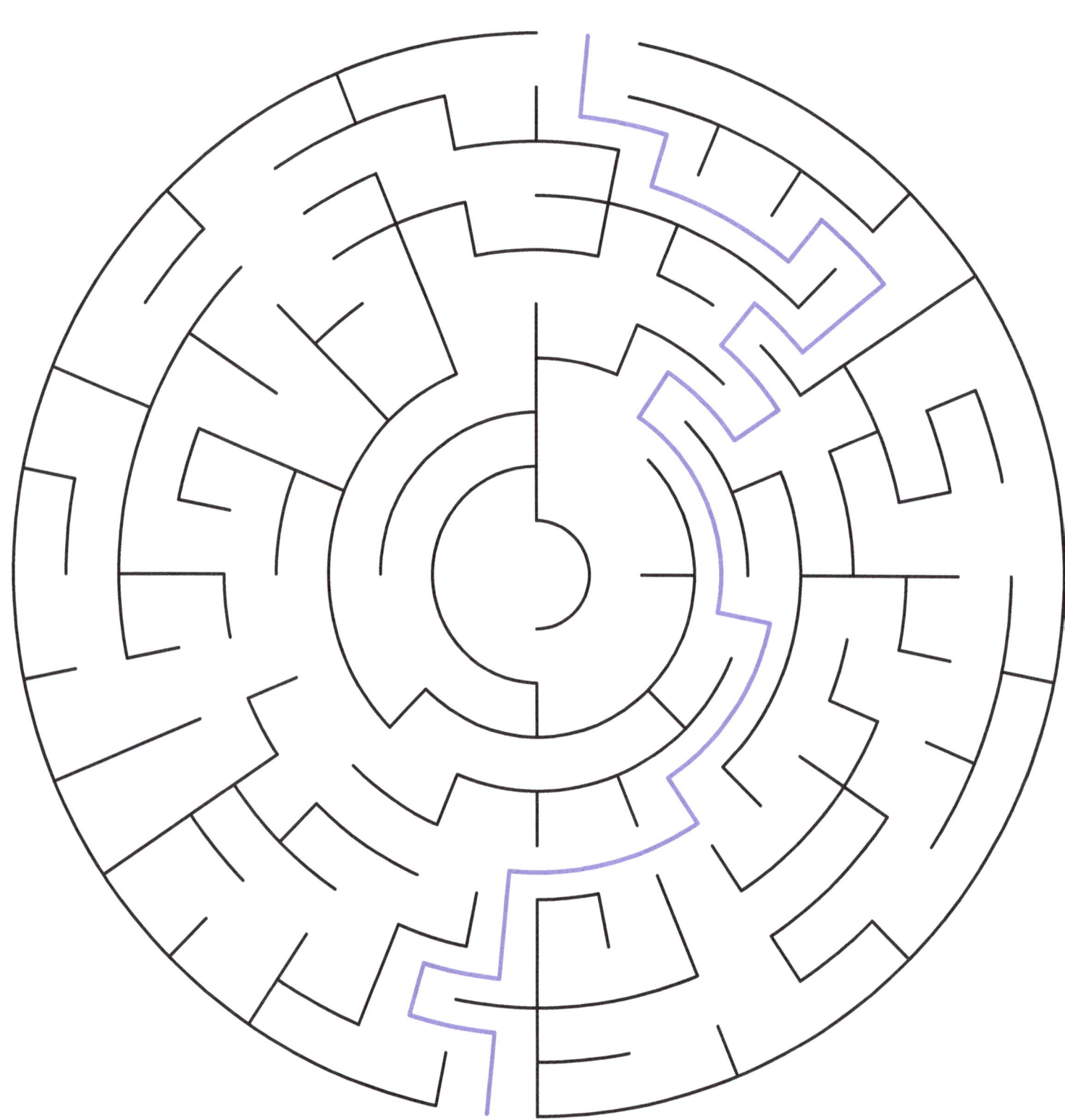

Maze Solution #30

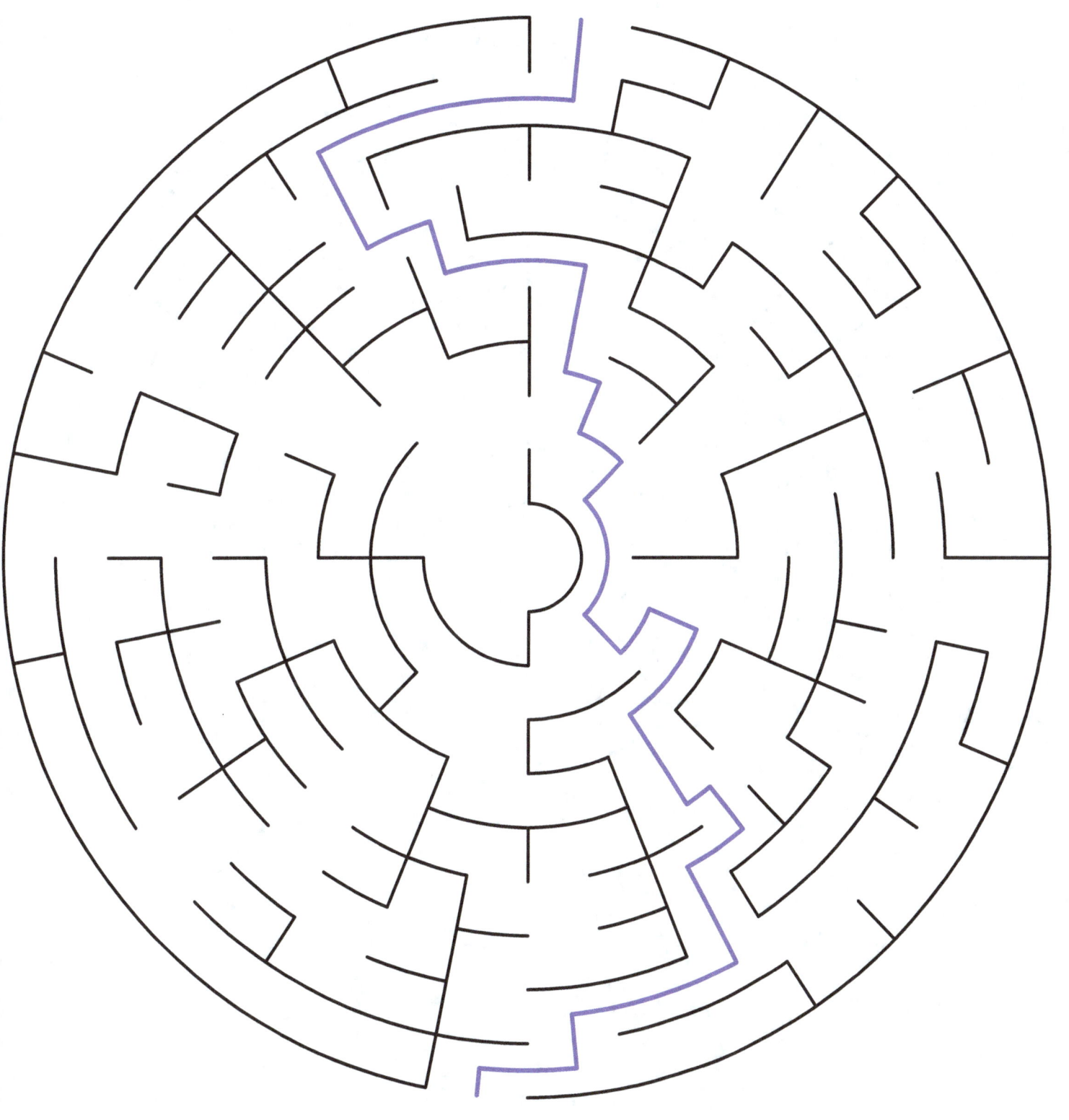

Maze Solution #31

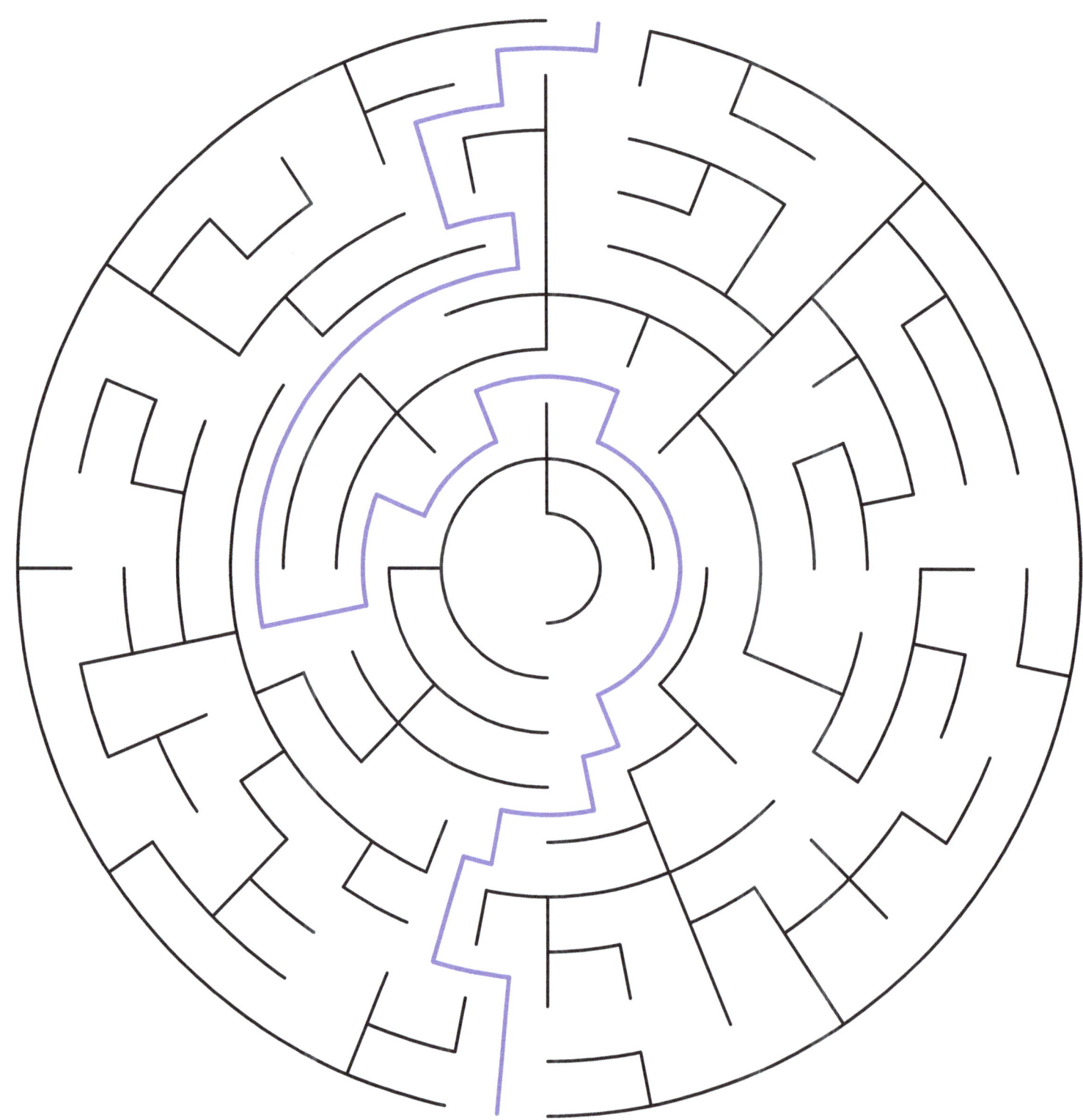

Maze Solution #32

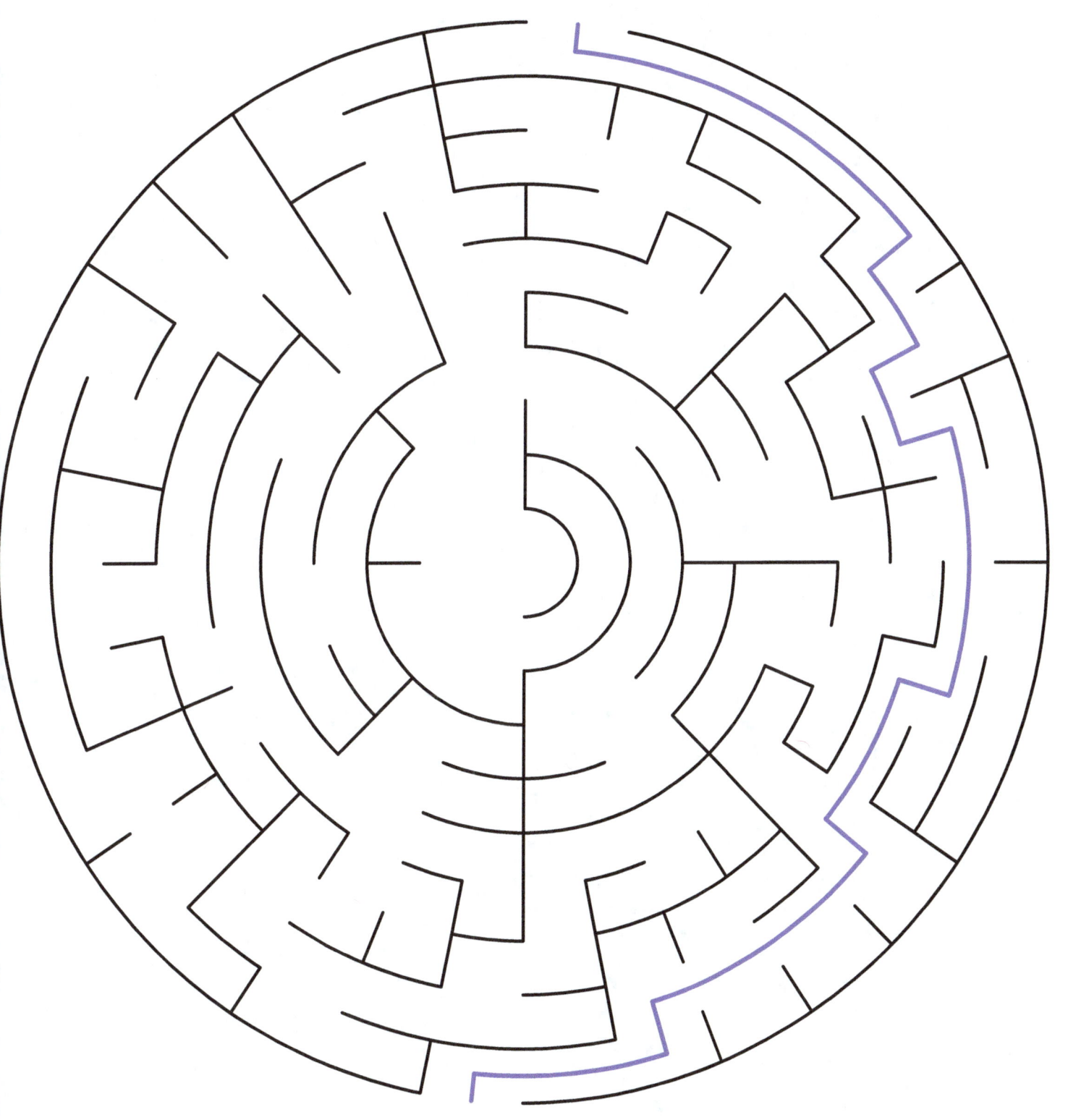